This book is the first in a series published in association with CEDR

Series Editor: *Robin Lovelock*

Forthcoming title:

VISUAL IMPAIRMENT: SOCIAL SUPPORT
recent research in context

Robin Lovelock

Changing Patterns of Mental Health Care

A case study in the development of local services

JACKIE POWELL and ROBIN LOVELOCK

Avebury

Aldershot · Brookfield USA · Hong Kong · Singapore · Sydney

Published by
Avebury
Ashgate Publishing Limited
Gower House
Croft Road
Aldershot
Hants GU11 3HR
England

Ashgate Publishing Company
Old Post Road
Brookfield
Vermont 05036
USA

A CIP catalogue record for this book is available from the British Library and the US Library of Congress.

ISBN 1 85628 333 X

Printed and Bound in Great Britain by
Athenaeum Press Ltd., Newcastle upon Tyne.

Contents

List of tables

Acknowledgements

Without the willing participation of the large staff group which *was* the Cosham Mental Health Service, this study could not have taken place. The team's membership changed considerably during the course of the research; our warmest thanks to everyone concerned. Similarly, if a number of users of the service - direct users, relatives, and referring GPs - had not freely given their time to speak with us in interviews, our understanding, and this book, would be greatly the poorer.

The evaluative study was commissioned and the funding agreed when the authors were based at the Social Services Research and Intelligence Unit, Portsmouth Polytechnic. The early stages of the work were carried out from that setting, but in the Autumn of 1988 both authors took up full-time appointments in the Department of Social Work Studies, University of Southampton, to which the research was transferred.

The evaluation was substantially funded from Joint Finance monies made available by Portsmouth and South-East Hampshire Health Authority, with active support from Hampshire Social Services Department. We are grateful to both agencies for this, and also to the many staff at different levels within them who helped us in a variety of ways during the course of the evaluation. Particular mention should be made of SSD staff based at the Cosham Area Centre, and to Paul Fuller, the department's resident statistician at Headquarters in Winchester.

Kay Murphy conducted a large proportion of the user interviews reported in Chapter 5, and carried out the first stage of analysis and writing based on the material collected.

Last, but by no means least, Jo Gooderham and her colleagues at Gower House have helped and encouraged us, not only to transform our research report into a book, but in formulating and launching the CEDR Series, within which it is the first of what we hope will be many titles.

Jackie Powell and Robin Lovelock
Southampton, May 1992

The authors

Jackie Powell is Lecturer in Social Work Studies and Associate Director of the Centre for Evaluative and Developmental Research (CEDR) in the Department of Social Work Studies at the University of Southampton. She is currently also Director of the department's postgraduate Personal Research Programme. Prior to taking up a full-time University Lectureship in 1988 she combined teaching and research through a series of specific appointments. Professionally qualified as a social worker, she has practised in a number of mental health settings. Her main research and teaching interests include evaluative research, the impact of changing organizational styles and patterns of service on professional practice, and users' views of health and social services.

Robin Lovelock is Senior Research Fellow and Director of the Centre for Evaluative and Developmental Research (CEDR) in the Department of Social Work Studies at the University of Southampton. He worked at the Social Services Research and Intelligence Unit (SSRIU), Portsmouth Polytechnic, from 1974-1988 and was Head of SSRIU from 1983 until 1988, when he moved to the University of Southampton as Fellow in Applied Social Studies. He has a particular interest in the methodology of evaluative research and has researched and published in a variety of areas of social/health care and services: physical (including sensory) disability, mental health, provision for elderly people, drug misuse.

Introduction

This book is about the organizational and practice issues involved in the process of implementing a 'community care' policy for people with mental health problems. It is based on the findings of an evaluative study of the implementation of one district health authority's strategy for the decentralization of its adult mental health services. The detailed research focused upon the work and experiences of a multidisciplinary staff team serving one local area within the City of Portsmouth.

Portsmouth has a large Victorian psychiatric hospital, St James', with a steadily reducing number of inpatient beds. Our main research interest however, like that of the local team whose work we studied, was the development of new-style services based in the local community. These included a residential facility, whose work mainly featured in the study through the way in which the staff based there had a substantial community as well as a residential role.

In current terminology, this book is therefore essentially concerned with aspects of the reprovision of mental health services, rather than directly with the run-down and closure of large psychiatric hospitals, which others have recently addressed in more detail (e.g. Wing, 1989; Korman and Glennerster, 1990). It is also primarily about the quality of services, rather than their cost and quantity.

Whilst the implications of Sir Roy Griffiths' report on the management of the National Health Service (DHSS, 1983b) continued to make themselves felt throughout the study period, the research reported here began before the appearance of the same author's *Community Care: Agenda for Action* (Griffiths, 1988), and data collection was complete before the passage of the NHS and Community Care Act 1990, which ultimately followed it. However, since the implementation of this Act remains a major focus for everyone concerned with social and health care, the concluding chapter of this book discusses the findings of the study in this present context of service development.

The decentralization process undertaken by Portsmouth and South-East Hampshire Health Authority in some ways anticipated changes now taking place more widely and involving statutory and voluntary agencies outside the NHS. A variety of readers may therefore find lessons for the present and future in this account of one health authority's pioneering venture.

Increasing attention is now being given to the evaluation of services, particularly in the context of new and changing forms of provision. This is to be welcomed. However, the approaches to evaluation most commonly used in relation to policy and practice typically overlook a number of theoretical problems. As Smith and Cantley (1985, p. 14) argue:

> [L]ittle is to be gained by pretending that the dynamics of pursuing and evaluating success are simpler than they really are.

We hope that this book will contribute to continuing methodological debate about evaluative research, and this opening chapter includes some discussion of the challenging issues involved. However, it is first necessary to set our case study against its broader substantive background.

The national context

The desire to provide care and services for mentally ill people in a community context rather than in large institutions has been an established feature of government policy in Britain for some time. *Better Services for the Mentally Ill* (DHSS, 1975) and *Health Service Development: Care in the Community and Joint Finance* (DHSS, 1983a) can be seen as direct forerunners of more recent White Papers and legislation, including *Caring for People* (DoH, 1989b) and the National Health Service and Community Care Act 1990.

In the 1950s, Britain was at the forefront of the move towards the liberalization of mental health services and the development of an 'open door' policy. However, local provision was uneven in both extent and quality, and services generally for mentally ill people were not afforded high priority. Furthermore, progress since that time has been slow and patchy, with the policy shift towards hospital closure and the decentralization of services taking many years to translate into practice (Korman and Glennerster, 1990).

A number of studies (e.g. Jones, 1988; Ramon, 1985) offer well-documented accounts of the development of community care in the mental health field. It is significant that such progress as has been made has been characterized by a general preference for encouraging incremental shifts at local level from hospital to district services, coupled with a view, held until recently by a majority of key professional groups, that community care is not radically or essentially different from hospital care (Ramon, 1985). The brief historical introduction which follows merely seeks to highlight a number of important general issues, which lie behind the local developments on which our case study focused.

A Royal Commission on the Law Related to Mental Illness, set up in 1954, recommended a shift towards care in the community, associated with a revision and extension of the existing powers of local authorities to provide for patients not in hospital. The Mental Health Act 1959 embodied much of the spirit of these recommendations, but it was essentially an enabling Act, providing a framework for 'enlightened professional action' (Jones, 1988).

The publication of *A Hospital Plan for England and Wales* (Ministry of Health, 1962) gave further impetus to both philosophical and political debates concerning the provision of care in the community for this client group. New measures for reducing the number of hospital beds were proposed in this document, although in what was effectively its companion volume, *Health and Welfare: the Development of Community Care* (Ministry of Health, 1963), only general statements were made as to the desirability of care in the community, with no specific guidelines for the establishment of community provision. This approach to deinstitutionalization, rather than decentralization, with little attention to the development of alternative local services, has had its critics (Sedgwick, 1982). However, based largely on the optimism and idealism of the 1950s, the prevailing frame of reference over the next decade was the caring and healing community.

With the publication of *Better Services for the Mentally Ill* (DHSS, 1975), some concern was raised over the still substantial numbers of long-stay hospital patients and the lack of alternative provision in the community. The commitment to community care was firmly reiterated and a blueprint offered for the development of a local psychiatric service, based on a district unit. In addition, both multidisciplinary teamwork and the need for high degrees of local co-ordination and co-operation between agencies were emphasized. The need for health and social services to work more closely together remained a prominent theme in subsequent DHSS publications (DHSS, 1977, 1978). The 1978 document noted that substantial difficulties had been encountered in inter-agency collaboration.

A policy based on the decentralization of services and collaboration and co-ordination between agencies to some extent encouraged greater involvement on the part of voluntary organizations in the development of local services. During the 1950s, MIND, first established in 1946 as the National Association for Mental Health, became an influential pressure group in the move for new mental health legislation, and was particularly committed to community care. Subsequently, MIND developed the dual objectives of lobbying for greater legal rights for patients and encouraging innovative projects. Along with other influential groups, including the Royal College of Psychiatrists and the British Association of Social Workers, it made a substantial contribution to the revision of the 1959 Mental Health Act and the further clarification of the rights of detained patients.

The Mental Health Act 1983, however, like the 1959 Act, had little to say with specific regard to community care. It gave no additional responsibilities to existing service providers, other than a requirement that local authorities appoint a sufficient number of Approved Social Workers (ASWs), who would have a vital role in considering alternatives to hospital care at the time of investigating a request for compulsory admission. More generally, relatively little consideration was given to the far-reaching implications for professional practice of a more locally-based approach to services, and MIND's (1983) suggestion for a new community mental health worker failed to receive the attention it deserved. The proposal could at least have served to initiate a wider debate around the issues of differing professional interests and the extent to which users could genuinely have more influence on the development of services (Beresford and Croft, 1986; Croft and Beresford, 1989).

During the 1980s there was growing public concern over both the cost and the organization and delivery of health and other public services. One dimension of this was manifested in the government's intention to introduce into the NHS the alleged financial and managerial efficiency of the business world. In February 1983 an Independent Management Inquiry Team, chaired by Roy (later Sir Roy) Griffiths, was set up to enquire into:

> the way in which resources are used and controlled ... so as to ensure the best value for money and the best possible services for the patient ... [and] to identify what further management issues need pursuing for these ... purposes.

This task was completed in the space of nine months and the outcome published in what at that time was widely known simply as 'the Griffiths Report' (DHSS, 1983b), and now necessarily as 'the first Griffiths Report' or 'Griffiths 1', following the same author's second major contribution to national social policy debate (Griffiths, 1988). The 1983 report referred to:

> a lack of a clearly defined general management function throughout the NHS,

and (p. 5) recommended that regional health authorities and district health authorities should:

> [appoint general managers] charged with the general management

function and overall responsibility for management's performance in achieving objectives set by the authority.

In June 1984, following Parliamentary debate and legislation, a DHSS circular was issued requiring health authorities to establish a general management function and to identify general managers, first in regional health authorities, then in district health authorities, and finally at unit level. By June 1985 most district general managers had been appointed, with the final regional general manager's post being filled during July 1985 (Carrier and Kendall, 1986). The appointment at each level of single managers, with a clear overall responsibility for setting and implementing service objectives, introduced a changed perspective into the NHS in a relatively short space of time. In effect, it took little more than two years from the time of the setting up of the Griffiths Inquiry to the implementation of its key recommendations throughout the NHS.

Around the same time as these overall changes in management structure were taking place in the health service, the House of Commons Social Services Committee took the initiative in conducting a survey of community care. This revealed wide disparities between rhetoric and reality (HCSS, 1985). Particular concern was expressed regarding the numbers of former psychiatric patients sent to prisons or left homeless.

A report by the Audit Commission for Local Authorities in England and Wales (1986) reported similar findings, adding the recommendation that resources should be made available to local authorities to enable them to develop alternative community services. Although numerous particular service developments and areas of innovative practice were identified by the Commission, they found that these remained patchy and that major changes on a large scale had not taken place. Difficulties and conflicts concerning collaboration between the two major statutory agencies involved, and power struggles both between different organizations and different professional groups, were also reported. The Commission called for an independent review of community care policies, along with a full consideration of possible strategic options.

The Government's response was to refer the matter to the NHS Management Committee, and to invite its Deputy Chairman, Sir Roy Griffiths, to prepare a report. The consequent investigations were rapidly carried out and *Community Care: Agenda for Action*, the second 'Griffiths Report', was presented to the Secretary of State for Social Services at the end of 1987. However, its publication was delayed until the spring of 1988.

Among Griffiths' main recommendations were the transfer of responsibility for all community care provision to local authorities (in effect to social services departments), and the resourcing of this by 'ring fenced' grants from central government. Introducing his report, Griffiths (1988, p. *iv*, para. 9) wrote:

> [C]ommunity care is a poor relative: everybody's distant relative, but nobody's baby.

The White Paper *Caring for People* (DoH, 1989b) followed 'Griffiths 2', albeit after an eighteen-month delay (see Chapter 7), with the subsequent NHS and Community Care Act 1990 appearing almost immediately and then being quickly passed through Parliament.

As this sketch indicates, rapid and substantial organizational change, and continuing national debate, constituted the general background context of the more specific local changes and developments in mental health provision with which we were primarily concerned in the study reported in the following chapters. The speed at which overall national changes in NHS management took place was one very significant aspect of this. Another was that despite the upheaval of major organizational change, the new arrangements brought opportunities for those health service managers who wished to do so to take a lead in the development of community-based mental health services (Ramon, 1988). The further substantial proposals for change which were soon to be on the horizon, specifically concerning community care, have presented a major challenge to social services departments and the voluntary sector as well as to the NHS.

It has also been noted that at least since the mid-1970s there has been a strong economic dimension in the thrust towards care in the community, intertwined with the professional and philosophical arguments in its favour. The period of rapid organizational change which we are still experiencing has also been one of severe financial constraint on the NHS and other public services. As Jones (1988, p. 44) argues:

> Present DHSS policy is based on decentralisation: finance is limited, and authorities are being told to take their budgets and do the best they can with them. At best, this may release some new energy and initiative. At worst, it may destroy even the existing quality of care.

The study

Background

In the 1950s, Portsmouth was regarded as one of several important and successful pioneering centres, which, as Jones (op. cit., p. 30) reports:

> impressed visitors from the United States by the range and variety of services, by the enthusiasm of the staff and by the way in which hospital and community interests were being brought together.

In retrospect therefore, it is perhaps not altogether surprising that three decades later Portsmouth and South-East Hampshire Health Authority continued its tradition of being ahead of its time, embarking, early in 1986, on an ambitious strategy for decentralizing both the organization and the delivery of its services for adults with mental health problems.

A number of area community teams would work with and alongside other service providers in their localities to offer a range of support. There were five defined areas to be served by these teams: three covering the northern, central and southern parts of the city itself, with staff members initially based on the hospital site, and two for the so-called 'county' part of the Health District, with staff based at a day hospital site some ten miles to the east. Area boundaries would be coterminous with those of Hampshire Social Services Department.

We were keen to undertake research alongside these developments, building both methodologically and substantively on earlier work which we had carried out in association with the same health authority's Mental Health Services Unit (Evans et al., 1986; Powell and Lovelock, 1987a).

A formal research proposal for a two-year evaluative study was agreed after meetings in spring 1987 with the Unit Manager, his deputy, and a representative of the consultant psychiatrists, and with senior staff of Hampshire Social Services Department concerned with mental health services at county level.

We agreed to take the developing service in Cosham, the northern part of Portsmouth itself, as the main focus of our study. It was said to be the farthest advanced, with its move away from the hospital into a community base imminent. It could therefore be seen as a 'pilot' for the other areas and would provide an opportunity to observe how one team effected the process of transition. By focusing on one locally-based team, the various dimensions of the process of transition could be examined in considerable detail. We would also seek to keep broadly in touch with developments in the other areas within the District, particularly within the city, so that the research could contribute to any general review of the Authority's overall strategy, and in particular help to identify key issues needing attention for its effective further implementation.

District Joint Finance was negotiated to support the first year of the study. Later, a further identical sum was made available for the second year.

Methodology

Aims The general aims of the study were to provide an analytic description of the Cosham Mental Health Service as it moved away from the parent psychiatric hospital to a community base, and to assess the impact of the changing service, both on its various users and on its immediate providers. Our research plan included a series of more detailed aims, which are set out in the following paragraphs.

Aim 1: To examine how the organization and operation of the Cosham Community Mental Health Team relates to the Health Authority's overall strategy for the transition of the District's adult mental health services into the community. This will be considered both as one among several attempts to operationalize a general philosophy, and in terms of the actual organizational and managerial links between the day-to-day service in Cosham, its sister teams as they develop, and senior managers at District level.

Aim 2: To describe and evaluate the overall nature of the Cosham Mental Health Service as a comprehensive community-based facility. Particular attention will be given to what might be described as essential features of such a service, namely the availability of a range of help, and its acceptability and accessibility to its users as it evolves over time.

Aim 3: To examine the various roles and tasks of the multidisciplinary team as they evolve in the provision of the service. The impact of the change in service base on staff will be of particular concern.

Aim 4: To explore the relationships and collaborative links established with other locally-based agencies and informal networks in the area. The relationships between the Cosham Community Mental Health Team and the local area centre of Hampshire Social Services Department will be of central importance.

Aim 5: To identify and describe the various categories of service user, which will include other professionals and voluntary agencies as well as patients and their families.

Aim 6: To assess, from these various 'consumer' perspectives, the overall impact of the service on its direct users, their relatives, and relevant professional and other groups and services.

Overall approach These formally-stated research aims, which guided the study and the subsequent analysis and presentation of its results, were derived from the specific objectives and underlying principles of the Health Authority's overall decentralization strategy (see Chapter 1). They also reflect a general view of service evaluation which we have developed in the context of a number of studies. We have come to characterize this approach, which evolved further in the course of the research reported here, in terms of its combined emphasis on 'pluralism', 'process', and 'partnership'. As the following brief outline indicates, our overall methodological orientation has much in common with the work of a number of other contemporary British and North American evaluative researchers.

Organizations, including those which provide social and health care services, are not homogeneous entities with clear and unitary goals; rather, they are made up of a variety of sub-groups with differing interests and concerns. In addition, social and health care services typically have a variety of users with differing needs: not only direct users and their families or other carers, but in a different sense professionals providing services complementary to that forming the focus of the evaluation concerned. In the context of service provision and evaluation, there are also a variety of other less directly interested persons and bodies: local councillors, taxpayers, the general public etc. The 'pluralistic' approach to evaluation (Smith and Cantley, 1983, 1985, 1988) is founded on these features of the real-life context of many care services; features which the more traditional 'experimental' approach, which has as its background model the clinical or drug trial, finds problematic, fails adequately to acknowledge, or seeks to circumvent, thereby limiting the applicability and usefulness of its findings.

A second general point, which like the first is not exclusively relevant to community-based services but is of particular contemporary relevance in that setting, is that where a service is new and evolving its organization and operation are necessarily in a state of flux, as its detailed goals and the means of attaining them are being worked out and specified. In this situation, description and interpretation are arguably more important than measurement and prediction (Buist, 1988, p. 74). The significance of this, and the importance of acknowledging the dimension of process in the design and conduct of evaluative research, has been emphasized strongly in the 'illuminative' approach developed by some educational researchers (Parlett and King, 1971; Parlett and Hamilton, 1972, 1977; Buist, op. cit.). These too reject the positivistic frame of reference which, through the influence of experimental psychology, has dominated their discipline's approach to the evaluation of innovations, and adopt instead an interpretive perspective on understanding change. The 'progressive refocusing' of key issues, characteristic of ethnographic research more generally (Hammersley and Atkinson, 1983), is an important part of 'illuminative evaluation'. The 'administrative anthropology' of Glennerster and his colleagues (Glennerster et al., 1983; Korman and Glennerster, 1990) also stresses the need for research in organizational and service contexts to be responsive to change. Any serious attempt at systematic evaluation of a development initiative must conceive not only the object of study but the research itself as a process.

Such strategic perspectives, which we share, have led the researchers adopting them to embrace and emphasize qualitative methods. In many cases an attempt is also made to combine several sorts and sources of information, often including quantitative as well as qualitative material. Any single method or source of data is likely to offer a limited perspective, yielding a better understanding of one aspect of a phenomenon and a less adequate one of others. In the inherently political context of applied social research, this may in effect constitute a bias towards one group or individual's views and interests.

This multi-method approach is commonly referred to as 'triangulation' (Denzin, 1970). Bryman (1989) has discussed its usefulness in case studies, such as that reported here. By bringing together a variety of data it is possible to overcome to some extent the limitations of a single method for describing the content and operation of a service and assessing its impact, and to take account of the process of development and of the several perspectives and often competing interests of those providing and those using the service.

The work of Guba and Lincoln (1981, 1989), again in the field of educational evaluation, emphasizes both the existence of a multiplicity of interests, views and concerns and the consequent plurality of legitimate criteria of success, and the ever-changing nature of the context of service evaluation. More explicitly than most of the writers referred to in the foregoing methodological discussion, Guba and Lincoln also share our own view that evaluative research which seeks to contribute to improvements in service quality is most likely to be effective if it is carried out in partnership over time with the several 'stakeholders' involved. In the study reported here we worked most closely with front-line staff and NHS managers. In certain parts of the research we also collaborated directly with social services staff; in others we sought to work in as egalitarian a spirit as possible with service users and carers.

We offered feedback throughout the study period to those most closely concerned with providing the service. An interim report (Powell and Lovelock, 1989a) after one year represented a more formal aspect of this, and was conceived as a working document, both for service managers and front-line staff and for its authors. In a sense this was part of the research process; it provided an opportunity to report on work in progress and to offer a reflective account of the continuing process of moving out and its impact on some of the various interested parties. The researchers were able to check their understanding of developments with those of some of the direct participants (McKeganey and Bloor, 1981). We have discussed this in more detail elsewhere (Powell and Lovelock, 1989b). The final report on the evaluation (Powell and Lovelock, 1991) presented, discussed, and drew together all the data collected, and offered an assessment of the development of the service over a critical two-year period of transition. Issues needing further attention were highlighted.

We believe that evaluative research of this kind, which provides a detailed and independent account of the development of a particular innovatory service, and assesses its impact from a variety of points of view, can directly contribute to improving services in one area. It is of more general relevance to a wider audience as a critical account of an example of 'good practice'.

Specific research methods Several methods or sources of information were used in an integrated way in the course of the study. Each was relevant in different degrees and combinations to pursuing each of the research aims listed above.

Material was extracted from a variety of documentary sources: various papers, minutes and other records concerned with the development of the overall District strategy and of the Cosham service in particular, together with case notes and related material.

We used observational methods, mostly semi-participant and of various degrees of formality. In particular, a range of meetings was attended, most importantly the regular team business and referral meetings, together with a number of staff workshops; staff were also observed at work in their several roles, both at their organizational base and away from it.

Routine statistics collated by the service and its partner agencies, especially Hampshire Social Services Department, were accessed. Other numerical material was generated by the research itself: for example from an analysis of 'the referral book', in which basic information was recorded in chronological order as new referrals were received.

A mixture of quantitative and qualitative information was provided by a series of 'logging exercises' in which staff recorded their activities, and via specially designed questionnaires exploring particular aspects of the staff team's professional views and practice.

We interviewed several groups of respondents: the immediate providers of the new-style service, a number of key actors in the overall management and development of the District strategy and in its integration with the work of other agencies, direct users of the service (clients and their families), and other professionals such as GPs (users of the service in a different sense) with whom members of the multidisciplinary specialist staff team came into contact.

Phases of the study We have argued that in evaluating services in transition it is necessary to conceive the research as a process, evolving over time and thereby reflecting the development of the service itself. It then becomes possible to explore key issues in increasing detail as the service develops and evolves over time, and to give due place to both the processes and the outcomes of change. In the present case, that of an innovative community-based service, the key issues were identified in general terms in our stated research aims as the essential features of the proposed locally-based service. However, the detailed factors affecting the successful implementation of the strategy could only emerge over time.

Our original research proposal acknowledged the lack of specificity of the stated aims and objectives of the service, which was appropriate to our own understanding of the nature of innovation in service provision and fitted well with the methodological perspective we have outlined. The proposal contained the following statement about the research strategy:

> Whilst we make no attempt at this stage to translate broad aims into specific objectives, it will be possible through the process of the research both to refine the more specific areas already

indicated, and to define other emerging ones for examination. Some changes over time may be identified, for example in the referral process, or in the extent of inter-agency collaboration. Thus the broad aims of the study provide a framework or overall strategy for the research, comparable to the *District Plan* with its service objectives, whilst retaining sufficient flexibility for incorporating both the anticipated and the unexpected as the service unfolds in one particular location.

We did not know at that time just how prescient those words were to become. A number of organizational changes within the service made it necessary to adjust the detail of our broad research plan; these changes would have shattered a more rigid design.

In early discussions it had been envisaged that the research would commence in the summer of 1987. However, it did not prove possible to secure funding until the autumn, by which time the proposed date for the Cosham service physically to move away from the hospital site had been put back until September/October 1988. It was therefore agreed that the study would begin on 1 January 1988, retaining the two-year timescale as originally proposed. This delay had some advantages, in that the research would now be able to span the revised period of transition.

Next, a restructuring of the overall management of mental health services in the District, crucially involving the replacement of the three Area Managers leading the separate local teams in Portsmouth by one City Manager with overall responsibilities, was announced shortly after the formal commencement of the study. In response we decided to give more research attention than had originally been envisaged to developments in the other parts of the city (Southsea and Central Portsmouth), particularly at the beginning of the study period, when we would be exploring the history of the decentralization strategy and those aspects of its implementation which had already taken place. In this way it would be possible to offer at least a limited comparison between the variety of detailed approaches adopted to operationalizing the new overall approach.

In the light of the somewhat fortuitous fact that the rescheduled move into the local community in autumn 1988 would fall at roughly the mid-point of our data collection activities, we had decided to phase certain aspects of the study so as to be able systematically to compare the service before and after its physical relocation. Thus, during the late spring and summer of 1988, when the members of the Cosham team were preoccupied with planning the moving out process, the researchers had parallel concerns. We had not adopted a formal 'before-and-after' research design, nor indeed prejudged in what ways, or indeed whether, the move as such would prove to be a critical event. Nevertheless, our overall approach and specific data collection activities were aimed during this period at providing descriptive accounts of the service in operation and of its users during the pre-move period, and recording the views of the team at this point in time, as a basis for a comparative examination of the developing service and its impact on staff and users over a longer timespan.

In the event, only a part of the overall Cosham service moved to a community base in October 1988, with an agreed plan that the residential facility, which remained on the hospital site, would move several months later. Thus the move, which for certain purposes could have been regarded as a single event, demarcating pre-move and post-move periods in the development of a decentralized approach, itself became a process: one whose own impact had to be evaluated, not least its impact upon the staff team providing the service. The overall study period now had to be reconceptualized as comprising three periods of time, which we termed the 'pre-move', 'partial move' and 'post-move' periods.

The detailed methodological consequences of this further turn of events are indicated at appropriate points in later chapters, where various aspects of the data are presented and discussed. It is important to indicate here that our overall research strategy remained essentially unchanged, being sufficiently flexible to be able to accommodate the necessary modifications. However, largely for resource reasons, it was not possible to collect data so as to compare the service on each of the dimensions we had selected during all three periods.

We had initially planned the time sequence of our research in several overlapping stages; however, these were altered by the events just reported. We present here only the broad phases of data collection as they now appear in retrospect.

Phase I: An initial period of observation of the day-to-day operation and the overall organization of the service, coupled with documentary work in relation to the history of the decentralization strategy and its various local manifestations.

Phase II: More detailed attention to the ongoing development of the Cosham Community Mental Health Service, focusing on the various activities undertaken by the members of the multidisciplinary team, including systematic exercises logging their activities in selected weeks and initial interviews with service providers. Further exploration via these interviews of the historical dimension of the development of the service and the initial impact of the move from a hospital to a community base from the practitioners' perspective. Examination, using specially-designed questionnaires, of team members' attitudes towards the development of community-based services and to working within a multidisciplinary team, and of their previous professional experience and perceived training needs. Early work on the inter-relationships between the team and other agencies.

Phase III: Collection of a range of baseline data concerning new referrals to the service during a six-month period. 'Tracking' these clients through the 'system' to the point of initial direct contact, drawing upon understandings developed during the initial stages of the study and using case notes and other sources. Initiation of data collection concerning mental health referrals to the local area centre of Hampshire Social Services Department, to elaborate upon the earlier work on the inter-relationships between the Cosham Mental Health Team and other agencies.

Phase IV: A second period of logging team activities. Collection of information concerning a further six-month cohort of new referrals. Follow-up questionnaires on staff attitudes and perceptions of expertise, interests and training needs.

Phase V: Interviews with key personnel involved in developing continuing care services, and group interviews with users of these services.

Phase VI: Interviews with service users, including some direct clients, their families, and a range of referring professionals, concentrating upon their perspectives on the overall impact of the changing service.

This sequence reveals in more detail the evolving process of the research. The various methods of data collection indicated earlier were used to differing degrees during different periods of the study, with particular sources of information being most important at particular stages. Broadly speaking, documentary and observational work predominated at the beginning, when the main task was to gain an overall understanding of the service. Key meetings and staff workshops were, however, attended throughout. Most of the statistical and questionnaire work, and the logging studies, took place during the middle period. These were designed to examine certain aspects of the service in some detail and over time. Interviews, particularly those with service users, were mainly conducted towards the end of the research, when the detailed issues to be explored by this means had emerged. The remaining task was then to bring the various sorts of data together and to relate the whole to the aims of the study, so as to offer an overall evaluation of the service as it had developed.

The structure of the book

Each of the stated aims of the evaluative study pointed to a particular area for investigation, relevant to the development of community-based mental health services. Decentralization, diversification, collaboration, boundary issues, and 'consumerism' are the dominant themes in this context, along with the central role of skilled professional practitioners.

The next six chapters present data focusing in turn on these areas of interest. Each chapter primarily relates to one of the research aims. Chapter 1 considers the organizational changes associated with the decentralization of the service (aim 1). Chapter 2 is concerned with the nature, style and diversity of the evolving community-based approach (aim 2). Chapter 3 focuses on collaborative links with other agencies, particularly those involving the local social services area centre (aim 4). The boundaries of the specialist service (aim 5), particularly in relation to the processes of referral and allocation to team members, form the subject matter of Chapter 4. Patterns of service use and the views and experiences of various 'consumers', including direct users, their relatives and GPs (aim 6) are presented in Chapter 5. Chapter 6 turns to issues of professional practice, examining the staff team's views about community-based services, teamwork, training needs, and priorities for service planning (aim 3).

Most chapters draw mainly on one source of data, although there are varying degrees of overlap. Each chapter pays attention to the evolution of the Cosham service over time; in most chapters there is some explicit comparison of equivalent data collected at different stages of the research.

Chapter 7 brings together the findings of the preceding chapters and reflects on the main issues and concerns of the Cosham service during the period of decentralization, assessing its relative successes and failures. Areas needing further attention are highlighted and discussed in the wider context of policy and professional practice.

1 Decentralization – Organizational issues

Introduction

To examine the relationship between the organization and operation of the Cosham Mental Health Service and Portsmouth and South-East Hampshire District Health Authority's overall strategy for decentralization, it is important first to explore the background and early stages of the transition of Portsmouth's adult mental health services into the community. Since a number of relevant decisions and developments took place before our research commenced, the following account of this stage in the process of implementing the District-wide strategy for establishing community-based services draws primarily upon documentation and interviews with key informants who had been involved in the early processes of planning and devolution.

This chapter first discusses the origins of the District's community-orientated approach to service delivery and the specific planning carried out in preparation for the major reorganization of adult mental health services into multidisciplinary teams based on local areas. It then examines the early development of the three teams which now together serve the City of Portsmouth, covering roughly the period from April 1985 to December 1987.

The chapter concludes with an examination of the main issues and concerns of the Cosham service as it prepared for and successfully effected its physical move away from the hospital site into its community base. In outlining the actual process of decentralization, we draw primarily on our attendance at the team's regular business meetings throughout the two-year period of the study, commencing in early January 1988.

The early development of a community-orientated service

National and local policy

The national policy objective of providing care and services for people with mental health problems in their local community had been reflected for some time within the Portsmouth and South-East Hampshire District Health Authority, with its well-established community psychiatric nursing service and the sectorization of acute services into local catchment areas.

The context for further extending the community orientation of mental health services in and around Portsmouth was provided in November 1983 by the publication of the District Health Authority's *Strategic Review* and its proposals for a pattern of services to be provided within the District for each care group by the year 2000. The Unit Management Team took the opportunity to produce a written response, formalizing many of their own and colleagues' current thoughts about redefining the Unit's philosophy and approach to the care of people with mental health problems. This group consisted of the Director of Nursing Services, the Unit Administrator and, as chair, the consultant who was also at the time Chair of the Psychiatric Division. Their document, entitled *A Strategic Review of Psychiatric Services* (1984), set out a philosophy of care for the Unit and included a statement of certain general principles which were seen as essential to the planning of a comprehensive psychiatric service for the future.

The key themes in these proposals were: an emphasis on the importance of staff rather than buildings and beds as the key resources; the development of an acceptable, accessible and locally-based service to meet the needs of individuals; and closer collaboration with other community-based organizations and facilities.

The document also highlighted the importance of careful planning and evaluation of these developments and the likely need for additional resources during the transitional phases, as well as acknowledging that the ultimate pattern of care proposed was not likely to be a cheaper option than the traditional one.

The overall strategy entailed the systematic development of a whole new range of community services throughout the catchment area, along with the simultaneous run-down of institutional services based on the St James' Hospital site. Whilst some service developments were already well-established in the community, the proposals emphasized the decentralization of the organization as well as the delivery of the service.

We noted in our Introduction that at the time these radical and extensive changes in the local service were being proposed, the management of the National Health Service as a whole was being examined by an independent inquiry team chaired by Roy (later Sir Roy) Griffiths. Among its recommendations (DHSS, 1983b) was the appointment of general managers at all levels within the NHS. Following Parliament's endorsement of Griffiths' proposals, Portsmouth and South-East Hampshire District Health Authority appointed a general manager early in 1985, and a general manager of its mental health services in October 1985.

Planning for devolution

With the introduction of these changes in overall management structure, the Unit Management Team was given responsibility to plan for the rapid changes required over the subsequent ten years to meet the objectives stated within what was now the District Health Authority's *Strategic Plan for Psychiatric Services*. In a paper called *Management Planning and the Communication System* (February 1985), the Unit Management Team argued that to develop and operate the new community-orientated service a different organizational structure was required. They proposed the development of five local community mental health teams, which would work with and alongside other service providers in their localities to offer a range of support. Three of these 'patches' would be within the City of Portsmouth, namely Cosham, Central Portsmouth, and Southsea, respectively the northern, central and southern parts of the city. Two further teams would cover the Havant and Horndean (part of East Hampshire) localities respectively, known together within the Health Authority as 'the county'. There were subsequently differences of view as to whether psychogeriatric services should be incorporated in an all-age patch system. (Although part of the Health District, the Fareham/Gosport area to the west of Portsmouth was not part of the catchment area served by St James' Hospital and is not discussed here. Mental health services for that part of South-East Hampshire operated from Knowle Hospital, near Fareham, and were administered by Southampton and South-West Hampshire Health Authority. This has been scheduled to change for some time and is now in the process of doing so, with Portsmouth and South-East Hampshire Health Authority assuming responsibility and developing a local multidisciplinary team approach.)

To assist the process of transition, a system of 'shadow management' was introduced, initially for a three-month period. Local shadow mental health teams were set up with the task of:

> undertaking an assessment of the major priorities for developing a community-based service in the relevant area [and] the steps necessary to achieve the required range of facilities, and to identify

a suitable operational base.

In many ways the setting up of these shadow mental health teams represented a natural process of evolution, with changes in organizational structure following developments in the service. For example, in the Cosham area a consultant-led team covering an area essentially coterminous with that served by the local area centre of Hampshire Social Services Department (called 'Portsmouth Area 1' at the time and subsequently 'Portsmouth North') was already in existence, whilst community psychiatric nurses (CPNs) were providing a community-orientated service and had established a number of community facilities in the form of 'contact clubs'.

What was new for these shadow teams was their wider membership. Under their terms of reference and constitution, each team was to include a consultant psychiatrist, a clinical nurse manager, an administrator, a psychologist, an occupational therapist (OT) and, where possible, a social worker. Each team was initially expected to meet at least monthly, to be chaired by the current sector consultant in adult psychiatry, and to have a formal agenda and minutes, which would be circulated to the Unit Management Team and all relevant wards and departments, as well as to the members of the shadow team itself.

The Cosham shadow team's main priorities

Like the other shadow patch teams, the Cosham team spent the early months of 1985 discussing a range of possible developments in the locality. There was general agreement that a base in the community, from which the service would be organized, was an immediate priority, and that ideally a site to the north of the catchment area should be sought. To cover the southern part of the area, the possible development of a base in the Battenburg Avenue Health Centre was considered.

Services for people with longer-term mental health problems were seen as the next priority, and there was a proposal to develop a travelling day centre, based on two or more sites, to provide low-key support within easy access of people's homes. This was seen as an extension of the work being done in the contact clubs at Cosham, Paulsgrove and Stamshaw, and a desire to involve local voluntary groups and the local social services area centre in these ventures was expressed.

Throughout the period to which we have been referring there was also continuous discussion about the need for residential facilities. The possibility of incorporating a residential unit within the proposed community-based mental health centre was considered, as was a proposal to situate a small number of assessment beds at the local general hospital. However, the identification in May 1985 of South and East Lodges - staff residential accommodation within the grounds of St James' Hospital - as available for alternative use, encouraged both the Cosham team and others to explore the potential of these buildings as an acute inpatient facility.

The consultant psychiatrist covering Cosham (also referred to earlier as chairing the Unit Management Team and representing the consultants' group on it) had for some time been keen to move his inpatient beds out of the main hospital. The identification of vacant property provided a possible means of making an initial move into the community.

Whilst this idea was being pursued by the shadow Cosham team, a second set of discussions was taking place elsewhere in the hospital concerning the possible development of South and East Lodges as a residential facility. For some time, several members of the Nurse Training Unit had been keen to establish a different type of residential provision, one which would give care in a setting as close to a normal domestic environment as possible. In siting such a facility in the local community, active links could be established with local networks and there would be an emphasis on developing a client-centred service. As well as challenging many traditional ideas about the provision of residential care, this venture also raised issues concerning the role of the nurse in the care of people with acute mental health problems.

In October 1985 two members of the Nurse Training Unit shared their ideas with the shadow Cosham Mental Health Team at one of the latter's meetings, presenting a paper which outlined a proposed model for the care and management of acute psychiatric patients in a residential unit. The minutes of the meeting noted the proposal as:

> a new radical approach for [the] integration of educational and clinical unit workings.

A great deal of discussion took place during this period, going beyond the shadow Cosham team. As one observer at the time commented:

> *It raised a lot of excitement, but also hostility, within the hospital. Many people felt threatened as professionals ... because it challenged a lot of our outdated practices and institutional thinking.*

The consultant for the Cosham area, looking back on that period, also made several pertinent observations about the difficulties which the team experienced in integrating various ideas from different sources in the planning of future services:

> *One of our initial problems was managing the thoughts that we'd had over some time as a community team of existing staff, who were working in the community, with something which was a bit different: ... a new-style residential unit.*

He did, however, feel generally positive, both about the idea and about the people involved, and not least because of the staff's enthusiasm and their commitment to developing an approach which challenged many traditional views and practices. He felt that it was right to support and encourage initiatives such as these, although tensions were created. As he explained:

> *One gets constrained by the way one looks at things. I think it probably would have been a less innovative service if I'd felt I had more control over it, simply because people have to approach it looking at it from different angles and different views. Although it has provided a lot of tensions over the two or three years I don't think these have been destructive overall. It has been beneficial, not least because everyone has had to modify a bit.*

Thus the development of a residential unit for the Cosham area represented a combination of several people's different ideas and concerns about the establishment of a less traditional form of residential care. Whilst a number of interests overlapped and there was common agreement on many aspects, for example on the need actively to seek a property in the local area, the merging of ideas involved was not entirely comfortable.

The implementation of the *District Plan*

Area Managers

By September 1985 the shadow mental health teams had largely completed their task of drawing up proposals for locally-based mental health services for the new Unit General Manager to submit to the District General Manager. There then followed a three-month management review from September to December.

The beginning of 1986 was a period of great upheaval at all levels of the organization, as plans for the decentralization of both the organization and the delivery of mental health services via a number of locality-orientated teams began to be implemented. In February five Area Managers were appointed, each directly accountable to the Unit General Manager. Regular Area Management Group meetings were also established, involving the five Area Managers, the Unit General Manager, and the Deputy UGM. The role of these meetings was to provide a forum for the discussion of Unit-wide problems or policy issues, to act as a working group during the six-month transition from a traditional to a community-based organizational pattern, and to work through different policies as required.

The Management Group noted that at that time in particular there was a need to implement the new proposals with considerable sensitivity and to ensure that adequate planning and discussion took place. Communication with staff, and team building, were seen as high priorities. This acknowledgement that the period was a time of major change was commented upon in interviews and discussions with us by many of those involved at the local team level, with feelings of uncertainty and confusion frequently being mentioned.

Of the five Area Managers, one took overall responsibility for psychogeriatric services and another for the 'county' adult mental health services, i.e. for the Horndean (East Hampshire) and Havant teams, both based on the Havant Day Hospital site. The three city teams were each separately managed, with their managers having varying sets of responsibilities. Two had additional responsibilities for certain District-wide services, over and above those for their respective adult mental health teams; the Cosham Area Manager also had oversight of Drug Dependency Services, and the Central Area Manager of Child and Family Therapy Services, Hospital Services and Alcohol Services. Although the Southsea Area Manager did not have equivalent additional areas of responsibility, it was noted that the development of the Southsea service in particular would need to emphasize provision for people with longer-term mental health problems, commonly referred to as 'continuing care clients'.

The updated *District Plan for 1987-89*, published in October 1986, outlined the overall strategy for mental health services through a number of key statements (p. 60):

> In accordance with Regional and National policies, the Health Authority intends to develop comprehensive community-based services for the mentally ill ...
>
> Services for the mentally ill will be based on multidisciplinary area teams for defined catchment areas. Within each area, it is envisaged that a mental health centre and residential rehabilitation facilities will be developed ...
>
> Services will be developed in close collaboration with Social Services, Education, and Housing Authorities, and voluntary agencies and, where appropriate, joint services will be provided ...

Underlying the development of these plans were a number of principles, which were stated as follows in the first edition of the Health Authority's 'official newspaper', the *Health Gazette*, in October 1986 (p. 4):

> The belief that people should have local services appropriate to their needs.
>
> The need for a flexible and sensitive range of services.
>
> Services which are easily accessible to clients, their families, and for GPs and other professional staff.
>
> Services provided in as normal a setting and style as possible, avoiding the stigma associated with the traditional mental

hospital.

The importance for clients to be recognised as individuals and maintain the maximum possible degree of dignity, independence and choice.

Establishing local services city-wide

In the early stages of implementation, working within the overall District strategy, each area team was encouraged to develop services in such a way as to take account of its particular local context. This variety of response was seen as both inevitable and appropriate by the planners and managers of the service, who stated that:

> A more flexible approach will ... be essential in view of both the resource uncertainties and the need to be opportunist when searching for suitable accommodation ...

As anticipated, the early phase of implementing the overall strategy was slightly different in each of the three areas making up the city as a whole. However, it was also evident from the outset that similar issues would have to be addressed in each area in establishing a community-based service. Each team would be operationalizing a general philosophy into a particular locally-based service, aiming to be widely accessible and to meet a broad range of needs. These needs would include those of people with longer-term mental health problems, whilst with the development of a community team as the focus for both the organization and the delivery of services, consideration of the role of the residential unit within the overall service would also be an important priority.

Whilst the evolution of services in the Cosham area will be our main focus in what follows, it is important to have an overview of the ways in which all three city teams dealt with equivalent issues, particularly during the initial establishment of the locally-based approach. This will help to provide links between the detailed account of the day-to-day operation of services in Cosham which we shall develop, and the wider strategic, managerial and organizational context.

The Southsea experience

As mentioned earlier, developing a service for the large number of people with continuing care needs living in Southsea had been seen as a major priority in the setting up of comprehensive local mental health services in that area. In addition, the Southsea Area Manager identified another pressing concern; the need to develop a team identity amongst the immediate service providers was seen as a first step to establishing a locally-based service. These two themes necessarily interweave in a brief account of the Southsea team's experience during the first eighteen months of its existence.

Team building As the first stage in team building, the Area Manager set up team meetings. These initially took place in one of the committee rooms at St James' Hospital - at that time the team had of course not yet physically moved out into the community. As the team's social worker explained:

> *[It was] an attempt to bring us more spatially together within the hospital, like a dry run. But it was too difficult because of lack of space, and so in fact we were still a very split team.*

Early in 1987 a decision was made to further split the Southsea 'community team' into 'acute' and 'continuing care' teams, in an attempt to ensure that the needs of the continuing care clients were specifically addressed within the wider development of a broadly-based local service. This decision to split 'the community team' presented difficulties for some of its members, in particular for the psychologist and the social worker. They each had a balance of work across the broad range of clients and so faced individual decisions regarding their team membership. For the CPNs the decision to work in the acute team or in the continuing care team seemed somewhat easier, in part because of the numbers of CPNs working within the service and the way in which particular individuals had developed their own work prior to the management changes.

In some ways the splitting of the overall team in this way, with the separate identification of an acute team and a continuing care team, specifically encouraged the development of a team identity on the part of the acute team, and this was reinforced by its subsequent move to a community base in Southsea, Cavendish House, in August 1987. This in turn encouraged closer examination of some of the key issues involved in putting a locally-based approach into practice; for example the team began to consider various ways in which their service might become more accessible and acceptable to its various users.

An open referral system began in Southsea as an initiative of the CPNs, who encouraged two general practices to make direct referrals to the team. Previously the CPNs had received referrals via the consultant. The social worker had also occasionally had work referred to her by the consultant, as well as directly by ward staff. Another new initiative, at a time when the traditional CPN service was still in operation in the remainder of the city and in the 'county' part of the District, was the introduction of an area duty system, which included a weekday rota covering Mondays to Fridays from 9 a.m. to 5 p.m. and a weekend rota. These two separate elements of duty cover each represented an additional aspect of developing a more widely accessible service.

The development of the continuing care team When the service devolved into local teams in April 1986, the Southsea Area Manager had been keen to address the needs of people with longer-term mental health problems. The Southsea area had already been identified as one of high priority in this respect, with substantial numbers of continuing care clients living in the many 'dwellings in multiple occupation' and rest homes to be found there. It is a long-standing and widely-held view that clients move and/or are transferred to Southsea from other parts of the city because of the greater availability of accommodation there, that staff working in other parts of the city contribute to this, and that Southsea has become something of 'a dumping ground' as a result.

The establishment of a continuing care team was seen as a way of ensuring that some resources were allocated to developing a service for people who previously had been the focus of little attention. This was achieved in part by a reallocation of resources away from the residential unit and into the building up of community services, in particular by the creation of a number of posts which together became the continuing care team.

Prior to the decentralization of the service there had been initially one, and then a further two, 'Special Projects Nurses', who had dealt primarily with clients with longer-term needs, particularly those who presented specific management problems. Along with a staff nurse responsible for organizing the city-wide 'depot' clinic, these three nurses had focused their work on ex-patients right across the city, although for the reasons just outlined most of their work was concentrated in the Southsea area. With decentralization, two of these special posts were 'relocated' to the other two teams in the city, ie those serving the Cosham and Central areas, whilst one, together with a nursing sister who had previously held a post in the District-wide rehabilitation unit, also located in Southsea, formed the core of the new Southsea continuing care team. Additional monies led to the creation of nursing assistant and OT helper posts, and of a post of 'Continuing Care Specialist'. An appointment was made to this latter post in September 1987, soon after the non-residential part of the Southsea team moved away from the hospital site. The post carried with it the substantial task of developing and leading the continuing care team; in addition, the incumbent was to identify particular areas of need, undertake extensive liaison with other agencies, and hold a small personal caseload.

Whilst the division of the Southsea community team into an acute and a continuing care team was important in raising the profile of work with continuing care clients, it also brought a need to ensure the integration of the community service as a whole. Many informal links were developed between the two teams, located in nearby premises in Southsea, the continuing care team being based at the rehabilitation unit referred to above. Contact mainly took place in the context of discussing the most appropriate allocation of work with individual clients. Initially there were some difficulties over the distribution of resources and facilities between the two community teams, with the continuing care team being seen as disadvantaged, for example in respect of available office accommodation. Many people would see this as in turn a reflection of the lack of priority given in the past to those people with longer-term mental health problems.

The relationship with the residential unit The Southsea community team was the first element of any of the three city patch teams to leave the St James' Hospital site. In making its early move away, this community team sustained relatively little contact with the residential unit serving the same population (Solent 2 Ward). This division in the service was encouraged by the Management Group's decision to make community developments in the Southsea area the main priority of that local service. As one team member suggested:

> *We're looking outwards and don't look back towards the ward very much. I think that feels like being left behind.*

By the end of 1987 the community team had come to feel a need to consider how they might work more closely with the residential unit within the overall Southsea service. Whilst they acknowledged that leaving the residential unit within St James' had given them time and a 'breathing space' in which to develop, the split in the overall service had become an issue needing attention. Addressing this was therefore to be a priority task, in particular for the newly-appointed psychologist.

Summary The Southsea team's main preoccupations during its first two years were with the development of a local and accessible service, and the establishment of a service for clients with continuing care needs. Underpinning these developments was the need for team building, which was also given substantial attention. The role of the residential unit, including its relationship with other facets of the locally-based Southsea service, was not given high priority early on, but it became and continued to be a focus of concern.

The experience of the Central area team

At the time when the locality-based approach came into operation, the Central area was identified as likely to be the slowest in developing services in the community. Only limited resources were available to the team, which was to remain on the St James' Hospital site in the short term.

As noted earlier, the Central Area Manager had additional responsibility for District Alcohol Services, Child and Family Therapy Services, and Hospital Services, the latter including the Brunel, or Intensive Care Unit. His initial task was to review a number of projects contained within the so-called 'Hospital Services', with a view to a reallocation of resources, particularly staff, from the institution to the community.

The development of the community team When services were decentralized in the spring of 1986, three CPNs moved from accommodation shared with a wider group of CPNs, to a small office adjacent to the residential unit serving Central Portsmouth (Solent 1 Ward). They represented the core of the Central community team, which over a period of time acquired additional members.

As the team gradually built up its resources, further developments in the creation of a more accessible service became possible. As within the other city teams, the establishment of an open referral system in April 1987 was an important part of this process. Following from this initiative the team began to meet together on a weekly basis, which was regarded by all members as an important means of developing a team identity and establishing and sharing a way of working together.

The first part of these team meetings was invariably taken up with a discussion of new referrals to the service, followed by a case review and then more general team business. The team, in describing the 'referral/allocation meeting', acknowledged the substantial contribution regularly made by the consultant psychiatrist, who provided a focus for the discussion and debate, which centred around the assessment of individual clients' needs. It was possible for each team member to make some contribution, and this encouraged the team as a whole to come to a shared view or team approach, with one person identified as the key-worker.

Lacking a full-time social worker for its first year, the Central team developed close links with the local social services area centre (then called 'Portsmouth Area 2', later 'Central Portsmouth'), from which a representative regularly attended the Central team's weekly referral meetings, both before and after the appointment of a social worker to the team in the summer of 1987.

As part of the reallocation of resources into the community team, one of the two long-standing charge nurses from the residential unit was invited to join it. He had earlier held a co-ordinator post in the Central area's 'shadow team' and, following a period of several months as Acting Senior Nurse Specialist/Assistant Area Manager, was confirmed in this latter post in November 1987. One primary aim of this transition was to encourage the process of team building, which was a particularly important task throughout the early life of the Central Portsmouth Mental Health Service. Team members did not come together in shared accommodation until the beginning of 1988, almost two years after the initial establishment of community teams, and all were still based on the St James' site at the conclusion of our research.

Despite their disadvantages, the members of the Central community team increasingly felt themselves to be an established group, sensing that in some ways their relative lack of resources allowed them to value those which they did have: primarily people. On the other hand, having few available resources meant that many of their ideas for developing community services could not be put into action. In many ways they felt 'in limbo', still firmly based in a run-down or dying hospital, but with considerable energy and enthusiasm for building up a community service.

Continuing care developments Interwoven with these team developments were other activities, more closely associated with the setting up of facilities in the local community for people with longer-term mental health problems. For example, two community-based clubs were established to replace the day hospital facility on the main hospital site. Also, one team member, whose appointment derived from one of the 'Special Projects Nurse' posts referred to in discussing developments in Southsea, worked mainly with clients receiving regular 'depot' injections at a local health centre.

The role of the residential unit Although some members of the Central area community team had a base physically very close to the residential unit, there was, as the CPNs observed, only very limited contact between the two parts of the service. However, during the latter part of 1987, both the community team and those working in the residential unit became aware of an area of overlap and difficulty in their response to clients requesting immediate help. There was a general recognition of the need to develop a more co-ordinated service to deal with personal callers, and it was agreed that staff based in the residential unit would undertake initial assessments in these circumstances. There were some early reservations about whether the residential staff were sufficiently skilled to carry out this task, and some concern that such developments would be at the expense of inpatients' needs. However, the system was introduced at the beginning of 1988.

The work undertaken in the residential unit was thereby broadened and thence overlapped more clearly with that of the community team. Not surprisingly, these developments encouraged the Central area team as a whole to consider how best to integrate all aspects of the service, so that the role of the residential unit in relation to the overall development of the community-based service became as much an ongoing issue within this team as elsewhere.

Summary Many of the issues identified as important for the Central team in developing a locally-based approach are similar to those raised in relation to the Southsea service. How these were addressed was determined to some extent by the decision to retain the Central team on the main hospital site in the short term. Despite some of the obvious disadvantages of a delayed move into the locality served, this also provided an opportunity for looking closely at the relationship between the community and residential parts of the service. The value placed on people as resources also appears to have been an important feature of this particular team's evolution.

The early development of the Cosham Mental Health Service

Having outlined some of the main features of the early development of the other two city teams, our attention now turns to the Cosham patch, which was the main focus of our overall study. From the earlier description of the Cosham team 'in shadow', it was evident that a major preoccupation even then was the relationship between the community and residential aspects of the total service. This issue remained of central concern throughout the early development of the Cosham Mental Health Service.

Residential and community resources Vinten House came into being in February 1986. It was described in the *District Plan 1987-89* (October 1986) as:

> a pilot acute (psychiatry) inpatient unit emphasising prevention, active therapy and community support to minimise the need for admission.

Six weeks later Vinten House became part of the Cosham Mental Health Service, responsible to the newly-appointed Cosham Area Manager. It was seen as an integral part of this service, both in providing residential facilities for the Cosham area and through its staff undertaking some work with clients in their own homes.

In the summer of 1986, about three months after the setting up of the District's local mental health teams, a service base for the Cosham team was established at North Lodge, a house on the perimeter of the grounds of St James' Hospital. As well as forming the main organizational base for the Cosham service as a whole, North Lodge was the common workplace of the Cosham 'community team', which was initially made up of the CPNs, the secretarial and clerical staff, the consultant psychiatrist, the social worker, and the Area Manager. The latter's responsibilities were reflected in the full title of the service she managed, namely 'The Cosham Mental Health Services and Drug Dependency Services'. Her deputy also had a dual role, reflected in the title of his post: 'Assistant Area Manager/Senior Nurse'. For a short period a psychologist shared the North Lodge base, but the particular post-holder had substantial work commitments outside the Cosham area and subsequently left the service.

As the first team to have an identifiable base away from the main hospital buildings, albeit still on the same site, the Cosham service was in that sense in advance of the other two city teams. However, with its residential unit, Vinten House, sited elsewhere in the hospital grounds, integration of the overall service presented many difficulties. As we have seen, maintaining a division between the residential and community facets of the service was possible in different ways for the other two city teams, and in each case this to some extent facilitated the development of a cohesive community team. Such a separation was not really an option for the Cosham staff group, since Vinten House itself had been set up as a way of providing a continuum of care for clients and with the aim of overcoming the traditional split between residential and community work. Having two separate work-bases did little to encourage the integration of what could easily be seen as two separate initiatives in the development of 'care in the community'.

Their physical location allowed the Vinten House staff team the space to develop what was an innovative approach, and a strong sense of teamwork was built up. The 'Vinten team' included two staff whose posts were partly funded by the School of Nursing and included responsibilities as clinical tutors, as service practitioners, and as joint managers of the House. The nine staff nurses, designated 'nurse therapists', were appointed to provide both in-house cover and additional work in the community.

During the first year of its existence, Vinten House and its staff faced a great deal of criticism, both within the hospital and from outside. Many of the comments made centred around the limited medical input involved there and the use of a range of social interventions. The latter were seen by Vinten's many critics as being employed at the expense of what they themselves regarded as more appropriate clinical approaches. Much could be written about the specific claims and counter-claims which were made, but it is important not to obscure two underlying areas of uncertainty: namely the appropriate place and role of a residential unit in the establishment of a comprehensive locally-based service, and the development of the nurse's therapeutic role.

In understanding the significance of some of the preoccupations surrounding Vinten House during the early months after the setting up of the patch teams, it is important also to remain aware of other concerns within the Cosham service, and in particular of the work involved in bringing the other team members together on the North Lodge site. With the need to develop appropriate systems for organizing the newly-established service, it was only too easy to continue to operate as two separate teams serving the Cosham area.

Team building The difficulties of team building and integrating the two elements of the overall service were further exacerbated by the dual responsibilities of the consultant psychiatrist and the Area Manager, each of whom faced substantial demands in relation to the development of a District-wide community-based service for drug misusers. This latter service, sited away from the hospital, in fact in Cosham itself, was in turn linked with regional developments in the drugs field based on the same site, in which the consultant also had a prominent role. Thus both the

'North Lodge team' and the 'Vinten House team' could be said to have lacked part of the substantial input they needed at a crucial time, and were thereby encouraged to take their own initiatives in developing the Cosham Mental Health Service.

As Vinten House staff began to develop their work in the community, some overlapping of activities with the North Lodge-based team was inevitable, leading to a degree of confusion both within the service itself and for other agencies in contact with it. This was to some extent exacerbated by the introduction of an open referral system, which enabled individual team members to take new referrals directly. In response to the recognition of a need for integration between the two facets of the service, a weekly referral meeting, at which all referrals to the service would be discussed and allocated, was established at the end of 1986.

A Liaison Group was also introduced at around this time, meeting for the first time in January 1987 and monthly thereafter. The formation of this group was a deliberate attempt both to bring together the diverse elements of the Cosham Mental Health Service and to promote a closer liaison between it and the District-wide service for drug misusers. As noted above, these two services shared the same manager, who felt that an exchange of the experiences gained in developing the two different community-based services could be mutually fruitful for staff and a source of ideas for further service development. The main aim of the Liaison Group's meetings was thus to provide a forum for such an exchange of ideas and information about the several individual elements for which the Area Manager (and the consultant) were responsible. Those attending would include the Area Manager and Assistant Area Manager, the consultant, social worker, OT and psychologist (when a new one was appointed), representatives from Highclere Drug Detoxification Unit, Vinten House, Northern Road Drug Advice Centre, and North Lodge. There would also be an administrative representative from the Cosham Mental Health Team.

Clearly, quite particular barriers stood in the way of team building for the Cosham service. It was impossible for the overall community team to become a more cohesive group without the issue of the relationship between those team members based at North Lodge and those based at Vinten House being raised. Given the actual number of staff involved, their different work-bases, and their different conditions of employment, 'sub-groups' were probably inevitable. How far they could be brought together in sharing the common task of developing comprehensive local facilities was in its particular manifestation a unique problem for the Cosham service.

An opportunity for promoting closer working together became possible with the resolution of another difficulty: that concerning the search for suitable accommodation for the service in the community. When the concept of Vinten House, and the idea of its becoming the residential unit for Cosham, had first been introduced to the shadow Cosham team, there had been general agreement that when the service moved out into the locality this should be as a whole service, rather than as separate residential and community facilities. There was also a strongly-held view amongst those who had been connected with the early development of Vinten House that an ordinary domestic dwelling, with a minimum of alterations, would be more in keeping with the expressed philosophy of the unit, which was to nurse people as far as possible in a domestic situation.

By the beginning of 1987, a number of alternative views had been explored about the most appropriate uses of mental health centres across the District. Should they be both organizational and service bases? Should residential units form part of them? There was a recognition within the overall Area Management Group that each local service would have to take developmental initiatives in relation to such facilities and resources as were available in its area. In Cosham, a site formerly used as an ambulance station was identified as a possible location for accommodation to replace both Vinten House and North Lodge. The decision to bring together the two separate parts of the service by a joint move to a shared location was specifically seen as a means of unification, as well as a practical solution to the problem of finding suitable accommodation.

Following this decision, the Cosham Liaison Group set up a working party from amongst its members, in July 1987, with a brief to prepare policies and procedures related to the development of the ambulance station site as a base in the local community for the whole Cosham Mental Health Service. This group was chaired by one of the two clinical teachers/joint appointees from Vinten House; its other members included a CPN, the recently-appointed clinical psychologist, and the senior secretary. One important piece of work undertaken was the production of a booklet giving information about the various resources and facilities provided by the service, including a 'Who's Who' of the staff, and explaining the system of referral then in operation.

Links with other services The Liaison Group took a number of additional initiatives to encourage closer links with other services. As an attempt to keep local GPs in touch with the various developments in the mental health service, a GP representative was invited to attend meetings of the group on a regular basis. A similar invitation was made to the local social services area centre, in anticipation of the particular need to jointly plan services for people with longer-term mental health problems.

Some collaborative activities with other agencies had already become established features of the service. For example, there were regular monthly meetings between social workers from the local area centre and some members of the Cosham team, mainly the consultant psychiatrist and the CPNs, who had been working in the locality for several years. The main focus of these meetings was on sharing information concerning individual clients and clarifying areas of joint work.

Continuing care needs In further recognition of the need to develop certain services in collaboration with other agencies, the Liaison Group established a second working party during the summer of 1987, to look at the needs of those clients requiring continuing care. It was chaired by the Assistant Area Manager, and its other members included the newly-appointed psychologist, the team's social worker, and a representative from the local social services area centre. The Continuing Care Specialist from the Southsea team, with her city-wide service development brief, also attended these meetings.

For the next six months this working party gathered together information about the probable nature and extent of need in respect of this client group in the local area, and about the range of provision necessary to respond to it. Much of this work was undertaken by the psychologist, who was given a particular brief in this respect at the time of her appointment. By the end of 1987 it was agreed that the continuing care working party, having identified many of the needs of this group, would now continue to work together in the planning and development of some form of day care provision in the local community. Both the continuing care working party, and that focusing on policies and procedures in relation to 'the move', were still in existence as the date for the formal commencement of our study approached.

Summary In contrast to both of the other two city teams, the first phase of developing the Cosham service was marked by a central focus on the need to build an integrated service, bringing together community and residential elements. Partly through historical accident, early attempts at team building inevitably encountered difficulties more easily avoided by the other teams at this stage.

In its attempts to develop greater accessibility, the Cosham service responded in broadly similar ways to the other city teams, introducing an open referral system and attempting to foster links with other local services. In its early attempts to address the issue of developing a better service for people with continuing care needs, the Cosham team engaged with other local agencies and organizations. Unlike the Southsea service it did this without creating an identified team of people to work in this field, although certain individual team members took on or maintained this area of activity as one aspect of their work.

Summary of the early development of the service

In this chapter so far we have sketched the origins and early development of a community-orientated mental health service in Portsmouth. There was considerable prior thought and discussion about the new approach at both District and Unit level, recognition of the need for major organizational changes as part of pursuing it, and conscious planning for their implementation. This fundamental rethinking, and the subsequent preparatory reorganization for 'going local', took place over a relatively short period, and at a time when the new, 'Griffiths-style' management structure was also being rapidly introduced into the National Health Service as a whole, bringing additional dimensions of radical change. The reflections of those who were involved suggest that the mid-1980s were experienced as a period of considerable upheaval and uncertainty, with the community mental health service which has emerged inevitably bearing the marks of this.

As later chapters will show, the pace of change was sustained throughout our study period. During the final phase of data collection and writing the Government produced its long-awaited response to the (second) 'Griffiths Report' (Griffiths, 1988), concerning 'community care', in the shape of the White Paper *Caring for People* (DoH, 1989b), and the subsequent legislation, the National Health Service and Community Care Act 1990, which linked this with the earlier White Paper *Working for Patients* (DoH, 1989a). The new national framework for mental health services which came into being in April 1991 will inform our concluding discussion in Chapter 7.

Returning to the early stages of the development of a community-based service for adults with mental health problems in Portsmouth, the means of implementing the new approach was and remains a District-wide overall strategy, allowing for local variation via patch teams with similar compositions. It was agreed that our research would focus on the development of the Cosham service, but we have included a brief account of early developments on the part of the other two area teams which, with Cosham's, provide mental health services to the 'city' part of the Portsmouth and South-East Hampshire Health District. We have indicated the way in which common issues arose in each area, with varying degrees of primacy, and how they were addressed in broadly similar ways, yet with differences of detail reflecting local factors.

In Southsea the development of a specialist continuing care service was a key feature, bringing with it the need to sustain an overall 'community team' identity embracing the 'acute team' as well. The latter's own sense of identity was in some ways assisted by the existence of the separate 'continuing care team'. The Southsea community team was the first to have accommodation away from St James' Hospital, and came to feel after a while that in a sense the residential part of the overall team had been 'left behind'.

The main features of the initial development of the Central Portsmouth service could be said to have been its relative lack of resources and the expectation that it would be the last to leave the hospital site. Like its sister service in Southsea, and for that matter the Cosham team, it had to be somewhat opportunistic in building up its community facilities. Nevertheless - and in part as a response to its difficulties - the team developed a strong sense of identity, based on valuing the people who have been its main resource.

Whereas the issue of the role of residential provision in the context of a community-orientated service only later became a priority concern for the Southsea and Central teams, this was the major influence on the early development of the Cosham service. We have shown that some of the reasons for this were essentially bound up with the fact that Cosham's initial residential facility, Vinten House, in the grounds of St James' Hospital, was one whose philosophy and practice itself challenged many traditional ideas about inpatient care and which embraced a community role for its staff. Added to this, the Cosham team was the first to have an administrative base away from the main hospital buildings - although still on the site. With each element having its own base away from the main buildings from early on, the integration of two overlapping but separate parts of the total service was the dominant theme. The central reason for the decision that our evaluation should focus on the Cosham service was that both residential and community aspects were to leave the main site together in due course.

The development of the local service

Introduction

By the end of 1987 there was a growing sense that the activities of the three local teams serving the city needed more effective co-ordination. The impending retirement of the Area Manager responsible for Central Portsmouth Mental Health Services provided an opportunity to modify the senior management structure, and with it the organization of the overall service. In January 1988, just as our research was formally beginning, a number of changes were proposed. These were seen by the Unit General Manager as:

> *[A means of] modifying the existing pattern, rather than a major organizational upheaval.*

The essential element of the planned changes which is of concern here, was that the Cosham team would be jointly managed with Southsea and Central Portsmouth teams as a city-wide service. The new Area Manager for the whole city was appointed from April 1988, having previously managed the Southsea service. The previous Cosham Area Manager retained her responsibility for Drug Dependency Services, to which were added the management of certain other District-wide services.

In this section, we offer a more detailed account of the overall development of the Cosham Community Mental Health Team as it planned for and achieved a key step in the complete decentralization of the service: the physical move away from the St James' Hospital site. We focus on the team's 'business meeting' over the specific two-year period of our study. These meetings provided a regular forum for the exchange of ideas and information between Cosham team members and the City Manager of mental health services. As we reported in the Introduction, for reasons which will be more fully detailed in this section it became necessary to modify our research plans to some extent and to divide our study of the developing Cosham service into three chronological periods: a 'pre-move period', a transition stage or 'partial move period', and a coming together or 'post-move period'. Our overview is presented in these terms and will provide a context against which to examine various aspects of the service in more detail in subsequent chapters.

The pre-move period

The evolution of the business meeting In the second part of this chapter we outlined the early development of the Cosham team and described the setting up of a Liaison Group at the end of 1986. During the following year members of this group, and the smaller sub-groups which it created, were actively addressing many aspects of the future move of the total service away from the hospital. By the end of 1987 considerable progress had been made towards bringing the community and residential strands of the service together in the planning of the new community facility. With a view to all team members together exploring some of these issues more widely, two workshops were planned for the beginning of 1988.

The first workshop took place in January. As it coincided with the formal commencement of this study it provided us with a useful introduction to the concerns of service providers at that time. The day had been organized to enable all team members to attend. Both the Cosham Area Manager and Assistant Area Manager were present, as were all three medical members of staff - two of the latter for part of the day only. Following agreement on a statement of intent or philosophy for the Cosham Mental Health Service, the main aim of the day became to identify and agree key issues for the period leading up to the move, then planned for some time in the early autumn. A list of points was recorded at the end of the day, as the basis for the second workshop a month later. These focused around the need to identify specific objectives and some shared goals, based on a clear understanding of individual roles and tasks within the overall team.

During the brief period between the two workshops the proposed management changes, bringing the three Portsmouth mental health teams together under a single manager who would be responsible for the whole city, were announced. Given the immediacy of these changes, both the new City Manager (previously the Southsea Area Manager) and the outgoing Cosham Area Manager attended the second workshop. Some concerns about the impact of these further changes in the service were expressed during the day. There was also general acknowledgement of the difficulties of translating a shared vision into everyday practice.

In the spirit of attempting to bring the whole team together, i.e. North Lodge and Vinten House staff groups, there was broad agreement to restructure the Monday morning meetings to allow more joint team activities. The referral meeting, which was already jointly co-ordinated, would be followed by a group supervision session, open to all team members. The Vinten House-based staff agreed to reschedule their business meeting to the afternoon to avoid any clash of commitments.

A little over a month later, with the City Manager taking up his appointment, a further change was made and a fortnightly business meeting for the whole team was introduced. Unlike the referral meeting and the supervision group, this was to be held at Vinten House, enabling a maximum number of team members to attend and providing sufficient accommodation for them. On alternate weeks, Vinten House would retain its own meeting to discuss day-to-day in-house business.

It was perhaps symbolic that the main item at the first joint business meeting was a final discussion of the building plans for the proposed community base, prior to work starting on-site. It was acknowledged that some modification to the original design was necessary in order to provide a specific reception area, more readily accessible from the front of the building.

At the third of these meetings, late in May 1988, it was agreed at the instigation of the Manager that the meetings would in future be held weekly and at a slightly later time, to give more team members - in particular the consultant and the social worker - the opportunity to attend. Each meeting would be chaired by the Manager, or in his absence by the Assistant City Manager, and would have an agenda and minutes. Over the subsequent five months, in anticipation of their move, the team's meetings reflected a number of issues, which not surprisingly were similar to those outlined in our earlier discussion of the preceding phase in the development of the service.

The role of the residential unit The major preoccupations throughout the pre-move period centred around the setting up of a small acute residential facility in the local community. This key issue presented itself in a number of ways, reflecting a range of concerns amongst the Cosham team and the wider service. For example, at the second business meeting a paper on *Presentations and Admissions to Vinten House* formed the main topic for discussion. Pursuing a policy of planned admissions to Vinten House between the hours of 9 a.m. and 6 p.m., the staff sought the opportunity to negotiate with the junior doctor on call regarding the appropriateness of any possible admission outside these times. This raised difficult issues about the respective roles of doctor and nurse, and the extent to which the professional autonomy of the former could be queried by the latter. These tensions were heightened by the views of some hospital staff that Vinten House operated an unusual and radical approach to both policy and practice. Discussions continued throughout the summer on these themes, which were acknowledged as of central concern by and for all Cosham team members.

Another facet of this issue was the more general question of medical cover, particularly that to be provided by the consultant and the junior doctor when the service moved into the community. The need to question some of the ways in which medical cover was provided across the whole Unit tended to be obscured by the assumption that this was a particular problem for Vinten House, rather than one facing any small acute residential facility seeking to function independently from a parent hospital. The relative lack of medical input to the Cosham service, due to the consultant's commitments to the District Drug Service, was also seen as a key impediment to any move away from the hospital. As the summer proceeded with this problem unresolved, concern grew about the likelihood of the Cosham team moving out as a single overall service.

Team organization for the delivery of the service There was evidence of progress on certain other fronts during this period, notably in the production and discussion of several policy documents. Firstly there was a statement of the aims of the Cosham service, its objectives and priorities. These were discussed and agreed by the team, following the presentation of a draft policy document by a small group derived from the working party on policies and practices. The development of a policy for a new duty officer system was also agreed. A significant aspect of this was that it took account of both the system of weekly duty then operated by the North Lodge-based staff, and the duty therapist system at Vinten House. The new system, introduced in August 1988, would operate on a daily basis and would embrace all team members who were not involved in the twenty-four-hour shift system; it would therefore include the Clinical Manager and the two clinical teachers/joint appointees based at Vinten House, as well as the North Lodge staff. Responsibility for daily communication with the duty therapist at Vinten House was to be an essential part of the duty officer's task.

Much of the discussion throughout this period touched on issues concerning the roles and tasks of individual team members. This was also the main item on the agenda for the first August meeting and discussion was wide-ranging. Questions were raised about the nature of the service itself, along with what staff resources, skills and expertise were needed to provide it. At this particular meeting it was agreed to hold a day workshop during the following week to explore these matters further. With the help of a facilitator, a number of issues were thereby identified and prioritized: medical cover, team identity, leadership and team members' roles. An agenda of items for discussion at subsequent business meetings was agreed and timetabled, with topics being assigned to individual team members on the basis of expressed interest.

During the next two months, several business meetings were taken up with discussion of a paper on the referral/assessment/allocation process. There was agreement that further work should be undertaken by the small policy group and a proposal drafted for subsequent team discussion. In acknowledging the need to look at how referrals were dealt with by the service, the team was also expressing some concern about the management of its overall workload. This was prompted partly by the imminence of the proposed move, accompanied by an expectation that referrals would increase, and partly by a growing sense that more resources had to be made available to meet the needs of people with longer-term mental health problems.

Our previous discussion of the early development of the Cosham service indicated that the needs of continuing care clients had been considered over some time. Information about a joint day care project for this group, with a proposal from the relevant working party of the Liaison Group that it be developed as a drop-in facility, had been discussed with the wider team in an earlier business meeting. The general topic assumed increased prominence during the late summer, when the Continuing Care Specialist was invited to attend to share her views on how services to people with longer-term needs could be substantially improved. One dimension of any development in this area was underlined: the need for identified team members to have a particular brief to work with continuing care clients. Whilst agreeing that this was a necessary prerequisite, the team was concerned about the possible implications of this proposal in terms of an expanding workload and the need to acquire the necessary skills to work in what a majority felt to be an unfamiliar area.

The service in transition

The partial move At the end of October 1988 the staff hitherto based at North Lodge moved to their new community base, Acorn Lodge, purpose-built on the site of the former ambulance station in Cosham. They left 'Vinten', i.e. the rest of the staff team and the residential unit as such, on the main hospital site, some four-and-a-half miles away.

The possibility of a split move occurring had been 'on the agenda' throughout the summer months, with the discussion largely centring around the still unresolved issue of medical cover for the community-based acute residential facility. This matter, which as we observed earlier is not simply relevant to Vinten House and the Cosham team, in turn raised broader questions about the still problematic relationships between the new-style general managers, appointed following the implementation of the 'Griffiths Report' on the NHS (DHSS, 1983b), and the consultants. It also relates to the changing role of psychiatrists in the context of the development of community mental health teams, and their particular contribution to the treatment of people with mental health problems. These issues are being more widely recognized as of increasing concern in the planned process of establishing community-based services (McKee, 1988).

With only a partial move of the service having taken place, what might have been anticipated as a single event became a process, and one whose impact itself had to be considered, not least its impact upon the staff team providing the service. Prior to the October move to Acorn Lodge of staff previously based at North Lodge, there were several indications that the team as a whole was becoming more integrated in its activities. For example, as we have seen, a policy document concerning the aims and objectives of the service had been drawn up and, more specifically, a revised and integrated duty officer system had been established. The split move inevitably raised the possibility of renewed divisions and fragmentation.

In recognition of these potential dangers, the need for a Co-ordinator of the community team, i.e. those moving away from North Lodge, was identified. Shortly after the move the senior OT took on this role. Her main tasks were identified as providing links with the City Manager and with other Cosham team members still based at Vinten House, and becoming an identified contact person for other agencies. Although there was no formal authority vested in the Co-ordinator's role, in many ways it was seen as complementary to that of the Clinical Manager, who had the responsibility of co-ordinating the activities of the residential unit.

At first, following the partial move, team business meetings were held at the two bases on alternate weeks. Subsequently, in an attempt to encourage the whole team to develop a more outward-looking or community focus, these meetings were held only at Acorn Lodge. Whilst the meeting day was changed in the hope of making it easier for residential staff to attend, the reality was that only the Clinical Manager maintained regular contact. This inevitably put increased responsibility on both the Clinical Manager and the Co-ordinator to maintain links between the separately-located parts of the service.

Priorities within the service Discussion of the referral/assessment/allocation process continued at the business meetings, uninterrupted by the partial move. The proposals outlined in a policy document on referrals and presented at a business meeting by the small policy group, were agreed by the team in January 1989. In many ways this policy document formalized the way in which the referral meeting was already operating as a system for both initial allocation for assessment and subsequent allocation for further work if appropriate. As an initial step towards identifying and managing the team's overall workload, a list of all the referrals to be discussed at each meeting was to be produced. There was, however, no mechanism for prioritizing these referrals in any way.

At a subsequent review of the new policy three months later, the possibility of prioritizing incoming work was again raised. Whilst the team acknowledged the need to make decisions regarding the relative urgency of each case, they appeared uncertain about whose responsibility it was to initiate such action. This lack of clarity was also reflected in the way that the second part of the meeting was operating; whilst some initial assessments were brought back to the meeting for further discussion, this process failed to operate routinely.

The uncertainty of the team in dealing with the allocation of new referrals to the service can be seen as but one part of a wider concern regarding the management of both the team's and each team member's workload, and about setting and changing priorities. The team also felt a need to establish closer working relationships with other agencies, particularly with GPs as the main referrers to the service. These related issues became the focus of much discussion at the business meetings, as the team began more actively to consider how to both communicate and negotiate with GPs concerning the making of 'appropriate' referrals to the service. At the same time, concerns were also expressed about the possibility of unduly raising expectations of the service and the possible impact of this on the team's overall workload.

Another significant development for the team was the formation of the Cosham Continuing Care Group in January 1989, representing a specific move towards developing services for people with longer-term mental health problems. At the same time this had an impact on the team's overall workload: more specifically on its ability to respond to requests for the assessment of new referrals.

Taken together, these developments implicitly raised questions about setting priorities and managing workload. Such issues are basic to the organization of teams and therefore central, not peripheral, to their existence (Øvretveit, 1986). This was evident in the way that the Cosham team spent much of its time during this period attempting to clarify its way of responding to the changing priorities of the service, whilst continuing to meet the demands of maintaining 'business as usual'.

Parallel and inter-related discussions about competing priorities were also preoccupying 'the residential team', i.e. those left at Vinten House, during this period. Their concerns over the relative balance between their community work, much of which involved the assessment of new referrals, and their in-house duties, mirrored the concerns of 'the community team' in responding to both new referrals to the service and continuing care clients. During this period the Clinical Manager was spending increasing amounts of time keeping the residential unit in touch with the community base. In recognition of this, an Assistant Clinical Manager was appointed, with the more specific task of co-ordinating in-house activities and preparing for the second stage of the move.

Moving forward together

At the beginning of June 1989, eight months after the initial, partial move, the residential unit moved from the hospital site into the community, thus uniting the Cosham service in a shared base. As a direct consequence of thorough planning and a considerable amount of hard work and commitment on everyone's part, but particularly involving the then Assistant City Manager, the coming together of the service was brought about with relatively little overt upheaval either to staff members or to service users.

Not surprisingly, over the first three months after joining their colleagues at the community base, the residential staff spent much of their time working out new policies and procedures for the day-to-day running of the residential unit. Of particular importance during this period was the clarification of the policy concerning emergency admissions and medical cover. Whilst the staff were already familiar with caring for residents in a domestic setting, the move to a purpose-built community base provided an environment which was new and unfamiliar in a number of ways. The residential unit was now operating away from the hospital site but in much closer proximity to other team members and the service's organizational base.

The most important staffing development at this time was the appointment of six support workers for the residential unit. The primary function of these non-professionally qualified staff was to provide additional in-house cover and support for the duty therapists, at the same time freeing the qualified staff to spend more of their time working with clients living at home.

These major changes in both the location and the staffing of the residential unit raised many questions about the future role of the nurse therapists, both in the unit and further afield. It also raised wider issues concerning the possible alternative ways in which the unit might contribute to providing care within the context of the overall service.

As we have already observed, the preceding phase of the service's transition - the partial move period - unavoidably provided different experiences and brought different priorities and concerns for those team members moving out into a new base in the community and for those left on the main hospital site. Not surprisingly it was a time of uncertainty, when the team as a whole experienced great difficulty in deciding how to respond to the growing number of demands being made upon it, both in terms of sustaining existing services and developing new ones. Coming together in a shared base served to increase awareness in the team as a whole of the overlapping nature of their concerns and the need to examine these together.

In recognition of the need for the whole team to consider how the different parts of the service related to each other, a forthcoming series of workshops initially planned for the residential staff was opened up to all team members. There was general agreement that within this wider context the team needed to look more specifically at how decisions were being made about limiting or extending individual or team workloads, and about setting and changing priorities. Although a substantial amount of work had already been undertaken on this, the team agreed to re-examine the referral/assessment process in order to attempt some prioritization of referrals and to develop a common assessment procedure. At the same time the team expressed a felt need for management support in the setting of its boundaries and in determining priorities.

Similar concerns had been pointed out earlier in the year: in our interim report (Powell and Lovelock, 1989a, p. 73) we noted:

> a need for the Cosham service to look more specifically at how decisions are made about limiting or extending individual and team workloads, and about setting and changing priorities. As Øvretveit, Temple and Coleman (1988) suggest, this responsibility rests both with senior management, in the setting of initial boundaries and objectives and defining basic aspects of the organisation, and with the team itself, in defining arrangements for managing its agreed workload. Achievements in these areas are vital for successful teamwork and thence to improving the overall service to its various users.

Summary

This outline of some of the preoccupations of the team's business meetings over what we have called the pre-move period, the partial move period and the coming together or post-move period, has indicated how the issues which were identified earlier as being crucial to developing a more accessible and responsive service, namely team organization and priority-setting, and the role of the residential unit, were being tackled over the extended period of moving away from the hospital. Throughout this time, the business meetings provided a forum where team members could meet together and, through discussion, begin to establish a shared team identity as the Cosham Mental Health Service. However, when only a part of the team moved out, meeting together as a whole team proved more difficult. Whilst important developments took place during the partial move period, most notably the setting up of the Cosham Continuing Care Group, it was really only when the service finally came together at Acorn Lodge that many crucial issues concerning team organization could be fully addressed.

Summary

In describing the early development of Portsmouth's District-wide service, and in more detail the Cosham experience during the period of our study, we have sought to convey some sense of the organizational changes which were taking place. The process of change has continued since the completion of the research. In the remaining chapters we turn to a closer examination of particular aspects of the changes and developments in the Cosham service over the two years of our study: 1988 and 1989. We attempt to highlight important issues in the process of decentralization, and to show how they were being addressed and to some extent resolved as part of an ongoing process of service development.

2 Locally-based services - Diversification

Introduction

The overview of the planning and development of the Cosham service presented in Chapter 1 has indicated its highly complex nature and the necessary bringing together of a range of facilities and activities. To describe how the overall service was operating and changing during the period of our study, and in particular to examine in detail how its various parts related and intermeshed, a two-part logging study was set up. A logging exercise was carried out during the pre-move phase and repeated after a settling-in period following the move, as a basis for a comparative examination of the service over time. All staff considered to be members of the Cosham Mental Health Team kept a record of their work activities during each of three separate weeks, roughly a month apart, in the period May to July 1988, and similarly during three separate weeks in the period September to November 1989. No logging exercise was carried out during the partial move period, when the residential unit remained on the main hospital site.

All staff members based at North Lodge took part in the first logging exercise. As shown in Table 2.1, this included all team members engaged in direct service provision (four CPNs, a senior OT, an OT helper, a clinical psychologist, a social worker, and the consultant psychiatrist), and the secretarial staff (a higher clerical officer, two part-time clerical officers and a part-time personal secretary). Not being direct service providers, neither the Manager nor Assistant Manager of the city-wide service took part.

Table 2.1
1st logging exercise - staff based at North Lodge

	Week 1	Week 2	Week 3
CPN1	/	/[a]	/
CPN2	/	/	/
CPN3	/	/	/
CPN4	/	/	/
OT	/	/	/
OT helper	/	/	/
Psychologist	/	/	/[b]
SW	/	St	/
Psychiatrist	/	/	/[c]
HCO	/	L	/
CO1	/	/	/
CO2	/	/	/
Personal sec	/	/	/

/=Completed logging
L=Annual leave St=Study leave

[a] Leave for two days of the week concerned.
[b] Sick leave for one day of the week concerned.
[c] Leave for one day of the week concerned.

Table 2.2
1st logging exercise - staff based at Vinten House

	Week 1	Week 2	Week 3
CM	/	/	/
NTh1	/	/	/
NTh2	/	/	/
NTh3	/	/	/
NTh4	/	/	/
NTh5	/	/	/
NTh6	/	/	L
NTh7	/	S	/
NTh8	/	/	/
NTh9	L	/	L
CT/JA1	/	L	/
CT/JA2	/	/	/

/=Completed logging
L=Annual leave S=Sick leave

All staff based at Vinten House, shown in Table 2.2, also took part: the Clinical Manager and nine staff nurses (more frequently referred to as nurse therapists), plus the two clinical teachers/joint appointees. In addition, although not shown in the table, a housekeeper and nursing assistant, who jointly contributed fifty-four hours, were involved during the first logging week.

It should be borne in mind that whilst many members of the team were engaged entirely on work associated with the Cosham Mental Health Service, some staff included here had additional responsibilities and spent some part of their week elsewhere. For example, the consultant psychiatrist was extensively involved with the District and Regional Drug Services, to the first of which both the senior OT and the OT helper also had some commitment. Two other doctors, an associate specialist and a registrar, provided additional medical input in the form of four outpatient clinics and medical cover for Vinten House. Neither of these two medical members of staff, who each had substantial commitments elsewhere, participated in the logging exercise, although many of the relevant aspects of their work were in effect recorded by other team members with whom they interacted, and are thus incorporated into our overall description of the service. Likewise neither the work of an additional clinical psychologist who provided two sessions at a local health centre, nor that of a second social worker who joined the team only during the third month of the first logging period, was formally recorded. Some of the Manager and Assistant Manager's contributions to the Cosham team, particularly the more formal elements, are also indicated in our general account.

Table 2.3
2nd logging exercise - staff based in community office, Acorn Lodge

	Week 4	Week 5	Week 6
CPN1	/	/	/
CPN2	/	/	L
CPN3	/	/	/
CPN4	/	/	/
OT	/	/	/
OT helper	/	/	/
SW1	L	L	/
SW2	/	/	/
JA	/	St	/
HCO	/	/	0
CO1	/	/	0
CO2	/	/	0
Personal sec	L	/	0

/=Completed logging
L=Annual leave St=Study leave
0=No information requested

For the second logging exercise, all staff based in the community office at Acorn Lodge (four CPNs, a part-time senior OT who by that time was also the Co-ordinator, an OT helper, two social workers and a joint appointee) and the secretarial staff (a higher clerical officer, two part-time clerical officers and a part-time personal secretary) participated, as shown in Table 2.3, although the latter group were only asked to log the first two weeks. Once again, neither the Manager nor Assistant Manager of the city-wide service took part; nor did any of the medical staff, although their activities in relation to the Cosham service were in effect indicated by others and are referred to in the discussion of the data.

All staff based in the residential unit, by this time located at Acorn Lodge, also took part in the second logging exercise, as shown in Table 2.4: the Clinical Manager, the Assistant Clinical Manager, and nine nurse therapists, plus a full-time housekeeper and five support workers.

Table 2.4
2nd logging exercise - staff based at residential unit, Acorn Lodge

	Week 4	Week 5	Week 6
CM	/	St	/
ACM	/	S	S
NTh1	/	/	/
NTh2	/	/	/
NTh3	/	/	/
NTh4	/	/	/
NTh5	/	St	L
NTh6	/	/	/
NTh7	L	L	/
NTh8	L	/	N
NTh9	M	M	/
Hkpr	/	L	/
SuppW1	/	L	L
SuppW2	/	/	/
SuppW3	L	/	/
SuppW4	N	/	/
SuppW5	/	/	/

/=Completed logging
L=Annual leave St=Study leave
S=Sick leave M=Maternity leave
N=No information returned

Although the participants in the second logging exercise were broadly comparable to those participating in the first, there were a number of differences which reflect staff changes over the time period spanning the move of the whole service into its shared community base. For example, whilst the number of CPNs in the community team remained the same, there had been a significant change among the particular personnel. A CPN who had worked primarily with people receiving short-term interventions was replaced by a CPN with a brief to work primarily in the area of continuing care. Other changes, representing a reduction in specialist inputs, involved the temporary loss of the clinical psychologist on maternity leave and a decrease in the number of hours worked by the senior OT. A second social worker appointment was, however, made during this period.

Staff changes in the residential unit between the two logging periods are more immediately apparent from the table; in particular there was the introduction of the support workers, who like the nurse therapists worked on a duty rota basis. Like the Clinical Manager, the newly-appointed Assistant Clinical Manager generally worked a five-day week.

During each of the six logging weeks, each team member was asked to fill in a daily log of activities, with a brief description of what these were, where and when they took place, and who else was involved. In order to make the daily completion of the logging sheet somewhat easier, a checklist of possible tasks and people with whom staff might have contact was provided. This was not seen as a comprehensive list, but rather as a helpful reference and reminder to the staff in the recording of their work.

The final selection of one week per month for the two respective three-month periods was made on the basis of being able to obtain logging information from as many staff as possible. Account was also taken of the Vinten House duty rota, operating on a fortnightly cycle, to ensure that each alternate weekly pattern was included at least once. As we have seen, some staff were excluded; otherwise, generally speaking, all relevant staff co-operated fully, providing the requested information unless on leave.

Analysis of staff activities by location

Where each staff member involved in direct service provision spends his or her time is of considerable relevance to understanding the organization and operation of the service. Tables 2.5 and 2.6 give a breakdown of the proportion of each person's total work time spent in a number of possible locations, both on the main hospital site and in the local area served, during the three separate recording weeks within the pre-move period. The consultant psychiatrist has been omitted from these particular tables, although not from the subsequent descriptive account. He supplied detailed information, but it is potentially misleading to compare a percentage breakdown by location of that varying proportion of his work time devoted to the Cosham Mental Health Service - as distinct from services for drug users - with time breakdowns of colleagues whose work

Table 2.5
Percentage[a] of their total working time spent at various locations by North Lodge-based staff - 1st logging exercise

	NL	VH	SJH	HC	CC	SSAC	HV	Other
Week 1								
CPN1	43	2	20	5	10	0	20	0
CPN2	43	0	0	0	23	0	20	14
CPN3	43	0	15	0	0	0	42	0
CPN4	45	0	0	0	2	0	53	0
OT	44	13	5	0	23	0	13	2
OT helper	44	8	0	0	36	0	12	0
Psychologist	54	0	13	0	0	0	13	20
SW	33	13	12	18	0	5	3	16
Week 2								
CPN1[b]	85	0	10	0	0	0	5	0
CPN2	28	2	15	0	8	5	20	22
CPN3	33	2	5	0	0	0	45	15
CPN4	40	10	0	0	0	3	47	0
OT	48	8	5	0	10	5	8	16
OT helper	42	8	0	0	33	0	17	0
Psychologist	50	10	5	10	0	5	0	20
SW			study leave					
Week 3								
CPN1	47	3	0	16	12	0	22	0
CPN2	52	3	0	0	20	0	22	3
CPN3	45	3	2	0	5	0	45	0
CPN4	40	5	0	2	0	0	53	0
OT	55	10	11	0	11	0	13	0
OT helper	45	9	6	0	23	0	18	0
Psychologist[c]	44	0	0	25	3	0	3	25
SW	35	10	17	13	0	0	10	15

a Figures in rows represent percentages of the total time worked during the relevant week by the team member concerned; e.g., if the week included one day's leave, the percentage is of approximately 4/5 of a full week. The consultant psychiatrist has been excluded (see text).

b Leave for two days of the week concerned.

c Sick leave for one day of the week concerned.

Table 2.6
Percentage[a] of their total working time spent at various locations by Vinten House-based staff - 1st logging exercise

	NL	VH	SJH	HC	CC	SSAC	HV	Other
Week 1								
CM	12	68	20	0	0	0	0	0
NTh1	0	64	14	22	0	0	0	0
NTh2	0	52	10	16	6	0	0	16
NTh3	0	86	0	0	4	0	10	0
NTh4	0	70	20	10	0	0	0	0
NTh5	0	100	0	0	0	0	0	0
NTh6	0	85	0	0	0	0	15	0
NTh7	0	95	0	0	0	0	5	0
NTh8	0	90	0	0	0	0	0	10
NTh9			annual leave					
CT/JA1	5	50	28	0	0	0	0	17
CT/JA2	0	30	70	0	0	0	0	0
Week 2								
CM	12	68	20	0	0	0	0	0
NTh1	0	78	0	22	0	0	0	0
NTh2	0	70	6	18	6	0	0	0
NTh3	0	80	7	0	5	0	8	0
NTh4	0	70	20	10	0	0	0	0
NTh5	0	85	0	0	0	0	10	5
NTh6	0	100	0	0	0	0	0	0
NTh7			sick leave					
NTh8	0	80	10	0	0	0	10	0
NTh9	0	90	0	0	0	0	10	0
CT/JA1			annual leave					
CT/JA2	0	14	66	0	0	0	0	20
Week 3								
CM	10	70	10	0	0	0	0	10
NTh1	0	90	0	10	0	0	0	0
NTh2	0	78	12	10	0	0	0	0
NTh3	0	94	0	0	0	0	6	0
NTh4	0	88	0	12	0	0	0	0
NTh5	0	95	0	5	0	0	0	0
NTh6			annual leave					
NTh7	0	90	10	0	0	0	0	0
NTh8	0	80	20	0	0	0	0	0
NTh9			annual leave					
CT/JA1	4	28	58	0	0	0	0	10
CT/JA2	0	40	50	0	0	0	0	10

[a] Figures in rows represent percentages of the total time worked during the relevant week by the team member concerned; e.g., if the week included one day's leave, the percentage is of approximately 4/5 of a full week.

Table 2.7
Percentage[a] of their total working time spent at various locations by community office-based staff, Acorn Lodge - 2nd logging exercise

	AL	RU	SJH	HC	CC	SSAC	HV	Other
Week 4								
CPN1	50	0	5	0	5	0	40	0
CPN2	31	4	12	8	30	0	10	5
CPN3	47	0	0	0	8	2	33	10
CPN4	(2)41	2	0	2	0	0	55	0
OT	62	0	8	0	13	0	13	4
OT helper	(8)45	0	4	0	42	0	9	0
SW1			annual leave					
SW2	(3)35	10	5	0	15	3	30	2
JA	(22)70	3	27	0	0	0	0	0
Week 5								
CPN1	(2)52	0	18	0	0	0	30	0
CPN2	(10)32	1	0	0	11	0	11	45
CPN3	(2)40	15	2	0	8	0	25	10
CPN4	36	0	0	2	0	0	62	0
OT	75	0	0	0	4	0	8	13
OT helper	26	10	2	0	58	0	4	0
SW1			annual leave					
SW2	(2)22	12	15	0	13	0	25	13
JA			study leave					
Week 6								
CPN1	52	0	3	0	0	0	45	0
CPN2			annual leave					
CPN3	37	8	8	0	14	2	21	10
CPN4	33	0	0	2	0	0	57	8
OT	62	0	17	0	4	0	17	0
OT helper	25	14	5	0	51	0	5	0
SW1	25	0	8	5	0	2	10	50
SW2	36	9	29	0	2	2	16	6
JA	(13)58	0	35	0	0	0	7	0

[a] Figures in rows represent percentages of the total time worked during the relevant week by the team member concerned; e.g., if the week included one day's leave, the percentage is of approximately 4/5 of a full week. Figures in brackets indicate the percentage of the total time spent at Acorn Lodge involving use of the interview rooms: this was not distinguished by all staff/each week. The consultant psychiatrist has been excluded (see text).

Table 2.8
Percentage[a] of their total working time spent at various locations by residential unit-based staff, Acorn Lodge - 2nd logging exercise

	AL	RU	SJH	HC	CC	SSAC	HV	Other
Week 4								
CM	(2)40	53	7	0	0	0	0	0
ACM	27	73	0	0	0	0	0	0
NTh1	(5)27	73	0	0	0	0	0	0
NTh2	(13)36	64	0	0	0	0	0	0
NTh3	18	79	0	0	0	0	3	0
NTh4	22	78	0	0	0	0	0	0
NTh5	20	80	0	0	0	0	0	0
NTh6	15	78	0	0	0	0	7	0
NTh7			annual leave					
NTh8			annual leave					
NTh9			maternity leave					
Week 5								
CM			study leave					
ACM			sick leave					
NTh1	(10)10	77	13	0	0	0	0	0
NTh2	10	79	7	0	0	0	0	4
NTh3	(4)4	96	0	0	0	0	0	0
NTh4	0	97	0	0	0	0	3	0
NTh5			study leave					
NTh6	0	96	0	0	0	0	4	0
NTh7			annual leave					
NTh8	(2)2	93	2	0	0	0	3	0
NTh9			maternity leave					
Week 6								
CM	(7)27	69	2	0	0	0	2	0
ACM			sick leave					
NTh1	8	90	2	0	0	0	0	0
NTh2	3	94	0	0	0	0	0	3
NTh3	(5)5	95	0	0	0	0	0	0
NTh4	0	92	4	0	0	0	4	0
NTh5			annual leave					
NTh6	(8)8	88	0	0	0	0	4	0
NTh7	(3)3	97	0	0	0	0	0	0
NTh8			no information					
NTh9	0	100	0	0	0	0	0	0

[a] Figures in rows represent percentages of the total time worked during the relevant week by the team member concerned; e.g., if the week included one day's leave, the percentage is of approximately 4/5 of a full week. Figures in brackets indicate the percentage of the total time spent at Acorn Lodge involving use of the interview rooms: this was not distinguished by all staff/each week.

was exclusively focused on mentally ill adults in Cosham.

Table 2.5 records the proportions of their time spent in different locations by the relevant team members based at North Lodge; Table 2.6 gives a similar breakdown for staff based at Vinten House. In presenting the data in this way, a difference in terms of contract as well as of 'home base' is implicitly acknowledged. All North Lodge-based staff worked a five-day week, as did three Vinten House-based staff, namely the Clinical Manager and the two clinical teachers/joint appointees. All other staff based at Vinten House operated on a three-shift/twenty-four-hour rota system, organized on a fortnightly basis and therefore involving each staff member in ten sessions on duty during each period. In theory, five of these duty sessions were spent providing in-house cover as the duty therapist and five working with clients in the local community. Whilst there are some noticeable differences between the three separately-recorded weeks of the first logging exercise, a broadly similar overall pattern for each is evident.

A similar analysis of staff activities by location was carried out using data from the second logging exercise; this is presented in Tables 2.7 and 2.8. In contrast to the pre-move situation, when the service's two locations were physically separate although both on the main hospital site, the two home bases were now within the same building, but with each maintaining separate access. The residential unit had its own front door and was completely self-contained, apart from a connecting door to the main office, which was kept locked. The community office was reached via a separate entrance, which also gave access to the room used by the group of secretarial and clerical staff. The community team, with the exception of the medical staff, shared a large upstairs office, near to three interviewing rooms and a consulting room. The latter was primarily used by the consultant psychiatrist. Also in this part of the building was a large room, known in recognition of the previous name of the residential unit as 'the Vinten Room', which was used for team meetings and similar sizeable gatherings. Thus whilst the community office was in many respects a direct replacement for the North Lodge base, there were now a number of additional interviewing facilities, available to all team members.

We shall now examine the data presented in the four tables on the preceding pages in some detail. Our overall aim is to give a picture of the day-to-day operation of the Cosham Mental Health Service as a whole, and to see how this changed over the period in which it moved its base from the St James' Hospital site to Acorn Lodge in Cosham itself. Our descriptive account of the service based on staff time spent at various locations must therefore pay attention to differences between the work patterns of the two groups of staff making up the overall team (as well as to those between individuals and sub-groups within each), and to changes in the typical weekly pattern(s) between the two logging periods.

North Lodge/community office at Acorn Lodge

As well as being the main organizational base for the overall service when the first logging exercise took place, in terms of clerical and administrative support, location of files etc., North Lodge provided office accommodation for all team members who were personally based there. Data collected for logging weeks 1, 2 and 3 show that these members of staff spent substantial amounts of their time at North Lodge, engaged in a range of administrative tasks and in informal contact with other team members sharing the same base. In addition, several meetings took place at this location, including the regular Monday referral meeting mentioned in the previous chapter, and a policy group meeting, generally arranged for a Thursday. The Clinical Manager based at Vinten House attended both of these meetings as part of her co-ordinating role. This largely accounts for the amount of time she recorded as spent at North Lodge, where other Vinten staff spent little time.

With the establishment of Acorn Lodge as the organizational base for the whole Cosham Mental Health Service, members of the team based in the community office for logging weeks 4, 5 and 6 recorded substantial periods of their time as being spent at Acorn Lodge, engaged in a range of administrative tasks and informal contact with other team members, similar to those activities previously identified at North Lodge. Compared with other team members based in the residential unit, the Clinical Manager spent consistently more of her time in the community part of Acorn Lodge, although during week 4 a high proportion of time was spent in this location by all members of the residential team, who attended a workshop in the Vinten Room.

The main observable change between the two sets of data is the greater evident variation amongst team members in terms of the proportions of their time spent at their base when this was Acorn Lodge than when it was North Lodge. These differences appear to reflect individuals' different patterns of work rather than particular professional perspectives. These variations will be explored further in the next section, in the context of an account of the day-to-day operation of the service.

Vinten House/residential unit at Acorn Lodge

The primary focus of activity at Vinten House was evidently providing twenty-four-hour care; this was reflected in the substantial proportions of their time which all Vinten House staff spent there during each of logging weeks 1, 2 and 3. Given her co-ordinating and liaising role, the Clinical Manager spent a somewhat lower proportion of her time in the House than did the nurse therapists, whilst the two clinical tutors/joint appointees generally spent much of their time elsewhere, particularly in the main hospital.

All staff based at Vinten House used it, rather than North Lodge, as their day-to-day organizational base. At Vinten House there was a small office which provided limited space for storing files and a place for staff to undertake administrative tasks or to use the single telephone. Although this office easily became over-crowded, it was nevertheless an important place for informal contact between Vinten House staff. It had a significant function as an operational base, but this was deliberately contained and circumscribed in an attempt to minimize the impact of the more formal aspects of the service on the essentially domestic setting being aimed at.

Excluding the Clinical Manager and the two clinical tutors/joint appointees, Vinten House staff members who were working in a given week spent on average between 80 and 90 per cent of their total work time actually at Vinten and providing in-house cover. For the three recorded weeks in the first logging exercise the average figures were 80 per cent, 82 per cent and 88 per cent respectively. During weeks 1 and 2 the House was providing individual supervision for one resident at risk of self-harm, in addition to its normal activities, and in both weeks one nurse therapist was either on annual leave or off sick (in which case some additional cover was provided). In week 3 there was no need for this heightened overall level of in-house support, but two members of staff were on annual leave, so other team members had to give priority to providing sufficient in-house cover and support.

Thus it appeared from our first logging exercise that with a full complement of staff, approximately two-thirds of total Vinten staff time was being found necessary to run the House. This was higher than the 50 per cent of time formally allocated for House duty. However, if there were special needs, or if any staff were absent, then a higher proportion of each working staff member's time was required to maintain adequate cover. Whilst week 3 may be regarded as more typical in terms of total demands on staff time than weeks 1 and 2, it involved a much higher average input from individuals because of staff annual leave. Thus the amount of time actually available for community work varied in accordance with the needs of the House, which were regarded as the first priority.

Whilst these comments about the balance of time-use amongst Vinten House staff are broadly justified by the first set of logging data, the actual proportions of time identified as spent in the House must be interpreted with some caution. Some work took place in the House with clients who were not resident; for example the group for abused women met at Vinten House in week 3, so that use could be made of video equipment. It should also be noted that whilst large proportions of staff time were spent in providing cover and support within the House, the duty therapist and others providing this undertook a range of tasks, many of which did not involve direct face-to-face contact with residents. For example, night duty offered an opportunity for catching up on administration, provided that this did not conflict with the needs of individual residents at a particular time.

When the staff of the residential unit moved to Acorn Lodge, a small office similar to that at Vinten House served as a new home base, and was used as an informal meeting place and a focal point of activity. The rough proportions of total work time spent in the residential unit at Acorn Lodge by those based there during logging weeks 4, 5 and 6 were similar to those indicated for Vinten House during the first logging period: on average between 80 and 90 per cent. Once again however, these actual figures must be treated with caution. With the introduction of the support workers, some changes in staff activities not necessarily associated with any change of location could be anticipated. Further exploration of this issue will be possible using the more descriptive data presented later in this chapter.

The relatively small proportions of their overall time which North Lodge-based team members spent at Vinten House increased slightly in weeks 2 and 3 of the first logging exercise, reflecting the introduction of a business meeting for the whole team which was held there. The senior OT and the OT helper recorded more time spent at Vinten House than did the CPNs collectively, representing their regular involvement with groups of current residents. Other individuals, for example one CPN and the psychologist, recorded significant amounts of time spent at Vinten House during particular weeks, for example in attending the Vinten review meeting or in seeing a client on an individual basis.

Of those staff subsequently based in the community office, some team members recorded regular proportions of time in the residential unit during logging weeks 4, 5 and 6, whilst others recorded very little. With the change in location of the business meeting to the Vinten Room, some reduction in overall time spent by 'community staff' in the residential base was to be anticipated.

Community locations

The major part of North Lodge-based staff's work with clients was undertaken out in the local area, in a variety of settings, including clients' homes. An analysis of the time spent by individual staff members at different locations during logging weeks 1, 2 and 3 revealed their particular regular commitments, for example in local community and/or health centre settings. There was substantial variation between different staff members in the use of community locations, reflecting personal style as much as professional differences. For example, two of the CPNs spent significantly larger proportions of their time working with people in their own homes than did their immediate colleagues. Another CPN spent a lot of her time in community centres, much of it in weekly contact club sessions with clients. A fourth CPN spent time at community centres running relaxation groups, and also time at the local health centre working with clients on an individual basis.

Overall analysis of the time recorded as spent at different locations during logging weeks 4, 5 and 6 by individual staff members based in the community office, revealed a broadly similar pattern of use of a number of locations in the local community to that found earlier. However, a reduction in the use of local health centres is noteworthy, and reflects some of the staff changes which had taken place, as we indicated earlier. The clinical psychologist and one CPN had been active users of this type of accommodation; neither participated in the second logging exercise. The regular time at a health centre location recorded by another CPN represented his attendance at the weekly practice meeting of one group of local GPs. Home visiting continued to be an important team activity, although again one varying with personal style and preference as much as with differences in practice between professions. The substantial proportions of time spent by the OT helper in community centre locations represented her extensive involvement in the newly-established drop-in centre.

Staff based at Vinten House on the whole spent less of their time working away from their base than did their colleagues from North Lodge. However, some Vinten staff were also already using a range of community locations at the time of the first period of logging, and these were similar to those identified for North Lodge-based team members. For example, several nurse therapists undertook work at the Cosham Health Centre; others regularly visited clients in their own homes. Vinten House-based staff spent markedly lower proportions of their time working in community centres and in patients' homes than did their North Lodge colleagues. However, work locations in the community chosen by Vinten House staff members again appeared to be a matter of personal preference and style of working. As already pointed out, time spent in these locations cannot be taken to represent the total extent of this staff group's 'community work' during the period in question, since some clients were invited to come to Vinten for individual sessions, whilst others occasionally dropped in to join the House community.

During the second period of logging, staff based at the residential unit continued to record time spent in home visiting, but not in using other community locations. This reduction in the use of community centre, and more significantly health centre, locations may be related to the availability and use of interviewing facilities at Acorn Lodge. This will be given further attention later.

The amount of time which staff spent at the local social services area centre was relatively small throughout our study period, although weekly variations are of some interest. During the first period of logging, the social worker had individual contact with area-based social services colleagues in week 1. In week 2 other North Lodge-based staff recorded time spent at the area centre; several of them attended a meeting concerned with the setting up of a jointly run day care facility for people with longer-term mental health problems. In week 3 an equivalent joint meeting was held at North Lodge. No Vinten House staff recorded time being spent at the area social services centre during any of the first three recorded weeks. During the second period of logging the amount of time spent at this location was also relatively small, even for the team's social workers. This analysis therefore suggests very little contact between members of the Cosham Mental Health Team and social services staff based at the area centre in Cosham. However, as we shall see later from the descriptive material provided by the logging study, there was regular contact with a representative from the area centre at the weekly referral meeting held at Acorn Lodge.

Other locations on the main hospital site

The bulk of the time which various staff spent during logging weeks 1, 2 and 3 at locations on the main hospital site other than North Lodge or Vinten House, was taken up by various teaching and learning activities, such as attending study days or teaching sessions at the Nurse Training Unit. That substantially higher proportions of their time was recorded as spent in this way by the two clinical tutors/joint appointees based at Vinten House, reveals the significance of their teaching roles.

For the second period of logging, any mental health units other than Acorn Lodge were included in this category, both those based on the main hospital site and those in other parts of the city. The major part of staff time spent in these locations involved either teaching activities or meetings, the latter frequently associated with the planning of future services for continuing care clients.

Other locations

A more adequate understanding of the range and significance of the activities recorded by staff and which we have classified in the 'other' category, and their distribution between team members, is afforded by the descriptive account of the week's activities given in the next section. However, certain observations on Tables 2.5 - 2.8 can be made here.

In week 1 of the pre-move logging period, the social worker and one of the CPNs were involved in a visit to another service out of the area. The significant proportions of time spent in other locations recorded during week 2 can be largely accounted for by the annual outing organized for a number of continuing care clients attending a contact club. The regular commitment of the psychologist to research activities away from the immediate locality on one day each week is also illustrated. The social worker spent considerable amounts of time at other locations; in week 3 these included the local Crown Court and Hampshire Social Services Department Headquarters in Winchester.

In the post-move period of logging, one social worker during one recorded week visited a variety of locations, including a social services family centre and the Crown Court. Other team members recorded time spent in a range of locations across the city, attending meetings frequently involving people from other statutory agencies and local voluntary organizations.

Summary

Analysis of the activities of staff based at North Lodge during the period prior to their move, suggests that whilst North Lodge was serving an important function as an organizational base for the whole Cosham team, it more particularly represented 'home base' for the 'North Lodge (or 'community') team', members of which spent a substantial proportion of their time there, carrying out a mixture of tasks. Many of these tasks were client-related - involving letter writing, case recording and liaison with other professionals. Other activities at this organizational base included both formal and informal meetings with other staff members, many of which involved discussion and planning of future service developments. Almost all activities involving direct client contact occurred out in the local community, at a number of different locations.

Overall, a broadly similar pattern of activities was recorded by this group of staff in the second logging exercise, following the move, with Acorn Lodge replacing North Lodge as the organizational base for the whole service. Whilst substantial proportions of time were spent at this location, variations between individual staff were more marked than before. Most activities recorded by staff based in the community office primarily involved direct client contact, which now took place mainly in people's homes or local community centres. There was a reduction in the use of health centre accommodation.

Staff based at Vinten House during the first logging exercise were spending substantial proportions of their time within the House, using it both as a day-to-day organizational base and as a service base. A lot of this time was used in providing in-house cover and support, and seeing non-resident clients on an individual basis. A range of administrative tasks was also undertaken at Vinten, and several meetings were being held there. The proportion of time spent by nurse therapists within the House varied with the changing needs of the group of clients resident at a particular time and with the number of staff on leave. Vinten House-based team members were also undertaking activities further afield, to a lesser degree than their colleagues from North Lodge, but in some similar locations to those used by the latter group: for example a local health centre and clients' homes. The two clinical tutors/joint appointees spent substantial amounts of time on the main hospital site, generally engaged in educational and training activities, although this kind of work was also undertaken by other team members, both Vinten House- and North Lodge-based.

Similar proportions of work time were being spent in the residential unit by staff based there during the second logging period. However, there was some indication of an increase in one-to-one work with clients, although whether this was taking place in the session room within the residential unit or elsewhere in Acorn Lodge was not always clearly recorded. Home visits continued to be shown, but work in other community locations, again most notably health centres in relation to the earlier logging period, no longer featured in returns.

Presenting data comparatively on where staff spend their time may tend to emphasize differences and divisions within the overall service and to underestimate the extent of areas of overlap and shared activity. However, this partial approach serves to indicate the substantial impact of where 'home base' is on the nature and location of a team member's activities.

Data from the first phase of the logging study clearly showed that significant differences in how and where they spent their time were closely related to whether an individual was part of the 'community' or 'residential' arm of the service. To the extent that the first group of team members worked a five-day week, whilst the second was involved in a twenty-four-hour duty rota, significant differences are only to be expected. However, in addition to the impact of this basic structure on staff patterns of work, the initial physical separation between the North Lodge site and Vinten House seemed to be reinforcing differences between the two groups which were relevant to the overall development of the service. Following the coming together of the whole service at Acorn Lodge, there was still a degree of physical separation between the day-to-day bases of the two parts of the overall team, with separate accesses to the residential unit and the office accommodation used by the other staff. Relative work patterns of the two staff groups in relation to location, as revealed by the second set of logging data, continued substantially to reflect the home base of the individuals concerned. One important new area of potential sharing during the period of the second logging exercise as compared with the first was the availability of interviewing facilities at Acorn Lodge which could be used by all team members. Unfortunately, however, the second set of logging data did not always clearly indicate the relevant specific location, as noted in Tables 2.7 and 2.8.

This analysis of staff activities in terms of location helps us to gain a somewhat clearer picture of the various dimensions of the overall service over time, and to see how each staff member contributed to the whole by undertaking a range of tasks in the Cosham locality. To explore important aspects of the service more closely, we must turn to a more detailed day-by-day descriptive account.

Weekly pattern of staff activities

North Lodge-based staff

Given that staff members initially based at North Lodge and then in the community office at Acorn Lodge generally worked a five-day week, their contributions to the service as revealed by the two-part logging study are best presented in the form of a composite or 'typical' week, highlighting any notable changes which occurred during the period studied.

General features A 'typical week' during the first logging period apparently involved some activities which took place on particular days and others which occurred throughout the week. Of the latter, the day-to-day routine administrative tasks should not be forgotten, as they provided the framework within which the service operated.

All the secretarial/clerical staff carried out a variety of tasks, overlapping throughout the day. These essentially involved receiving telephone calls, dealing with initial enquiries, and undertaking a range of general office duties. All secretarial/clerical staff had considerable contact with other members of the overall team, with those members who were themselves based at North Lodge figuring more frequently. There was a great deal of coming and going during the day, as various staff returned to base to collect and deal with messages taken on their behalf.

Some administrative tasks were specifically the responsibility of one individual; for example one clerical officer had the task of recording all admissions and discharges to Vinten House, which involved her in daily contact with some Vinten House staff. During the first week of recording activities, the higher clerical officer was in the process of delegating a number of tasks to a newly-appointed clerical officer. Recording all new referrals to the service and attending the weekly referral meeting were tasks undertaken by this clerical officer during the second and third logged weeks. Whilst the higher clerical officer had the main responsibility for recording all 'Körner information' collected by the team, she was helped in this task by the part-time personal secretary. Although there was a very low recorded incidence of personal callers, all the secretarial/clerical staff had some telephone contact with clients.

Overall, the general features of a typical week remained substantially the same over the whole period studied. All the secretarial/clerical staff carried out a variety of tasks, which overlapped throughout the day. Whilst in the first logging exercise there was evidence of administrative tasks being more specifically the responsibility of one individual, in the second period of logging there appeared to be greater overlapping and sharing of tasks. For example, whilst recording all the new referrals to the service remained an important task for one clerical officer, she no longer attended the weekly referral meeting. However, she liaised a great deal with the duty officer in the preparation of material prior to this weekly event. The coming together of the two previously separated bases at a shared physical location was important in promoting areas of overlap between the organizational and substantive aspects of the service. Slightly more recorded incidents of personal callers were indicated in the second logging exercise, involving the secretarial/clerical staff in increased direct contact with clients.

Alongside the day-to-day activities of the secretarial and clerical staff were the tasks undertaken by those direct service providers also based initially at North Lodge and subsequently in the community office at Acorn Lodge. The workloads of these team members included a range of administrative tasks, undertaken throughout the week and occupying a large part of the substantial amount of time which they spent at their home base. North Lodge had a minimal function as a service base, other than its occasional use by the consultant psychiatrist for seeing a number of clients as outpatients. Acorn Lodge has some accommodation available for seeing clients, but this was used relatively little by these particular staff members. However, a considerable amount of telephone contact with clients, and with other professional workers, was recorded in each of the three logging weeks of the pre-move period and similarly during the post-move logging exercise.

With the exclusion of the medical staff, those team members directly providing the service and based at North Lodge during the pre-move period maintained a weekday duty system to deal with urgent requests for help. The psychologist, a CPN and the senior OT respectively were the duty officers for the first, second and third recorded weeks of logging. By the time of the second logging exercise, a daily duty rota had been introduced. The tasks associated with being on duty did not generally appear to impact significantly upon the regular activities of the duty officers, and are reported below as part of the day-to-day activities of particular team members as appropriate.

As we saw earlier from an analysis of their activities by location, a significant part of the working time of team members based first at North Lodge and later in the community office at Acorn Lodge, was spent out in the local community. Whilst domiciliary visits were made throughout the week, other important activities took place less frequently, but on particular days. These aspects of these team members' work are best described as they occurred during our constructed 'typical week'. Data from the pre-move logging exercise have been used to provide a basic descriptive account of each day's activities. This is followed by an update based on data from the post-move logging exercise, noting any observable changes over time.

Monday In the pre-move period, the first day of the week was dominated by a series of regular meetings, the first of which was the referral meeting, held at North Lodge. This was generally attended by those team members based at North Lodge: the CPNs, senior OT, OT helper, psychologist, social worker and consultant psychiatrist, together with one of the administrative staff, whose task it was to present basic information about all referrals made to the service during the previous week. The Clinical Manager from Vinten House also attended these meetings, occasionally accompanied by another member of the Vinten House staff or a student nurse. The main purpose of the meeting was to allocate each new referral to a team member for further assessment.

Both before and after this meeting, individual team members did some planning and preparation for the forthcoming week's activities, discussed events of the previous week, and generally exchanged information. Coming to the referral meeting also provided an opportunity for staff to get together informally, particularly with the consultant psychiatrist, to discuss both individual clients and administrative issues not dealt with in the meeting itself.

The referral meeting was followed by a group supervision session, which was usually attended by all members of the North Lodge staff group except the consultant, and by the Vinten House Clinical Manager. These sessions were used in several ways: for example, in general discussion of various workload issues, or in the presentation of a particular case for group consideration. In week 3 of logging, one team member whose work was discussed in this way recorded the session as helpful in terms of:

> *[being] given suggestions and ideas by other members of the team.*

For most North Lodge team members, the remainder of Monday morning was spent carrying out various administrative tasks, some of which were generated from the earlier meetings. The social worker attended a regular meeting with other members of the mental health social work team. These meetings were usually chaired by the Assistant Social Work Manager, who was based within the main hospital. The consultant psychiatrist spent most of his morning, after the referral meeting, seeing outpatients at North Lodge, before attending a regular weekly consultants' meeting in the main hospital. Two other outpatient clinics were also generally held on Monday mornings at the local general hospital, and a clinical psychology session took place at a local health centre.

By the second week of logging, a new meeting, variously called the 'management meeting', 'business meeting' or 'team meeting', had been introduced, taking place during the middle part of the day. This was usually chaired by the Manager, or in his absence by the Assistant Manager, and was attended by all the North Lodge team members and several of those based at Vinten House. It provided an opportunity for as many team members as possible to get together to discuss wider 'team issues'.

This business meeting was then followed by the weekly Vinten House review meeting, attended regularly by several Vinten House staff and on some occasions by other team members based at North Lodge. The consultant psychiatrist, when other commitments allowed, also attended both this meeting and the earlier business meeting, along with the junior doctor. At the review meeting, the needs of those people currently resident in Vinten House were discussed. As on earlier occasions during the day, there were also opportunities for individual staff members to discuss informally the care and management of various clients. After this meeting the consultant psychiatrist generally went on to complete his day with work for the District and Regional Drug Services, based at the Northern Road Clinic in Cosham.

An important feature on Monday afternoons was the contact club held in a church hall in the Cosham area. This was regularly attended by one CPN and a volunteer, and on some occasions by other team members, as in week 2 when the OT helper was present. This additional input enabled the CPN to use her time at the club more flexibly; for example, in the third recorded week she initially spent some time with the whole group, helping the volunteer and club members to set up and organize a games session for the afternoon, before seeing some clients on an individual basis.

The other CPNs carried out home visits during the afternoon, whilst other team members, such as the senior OT, spent the time at North Lodge, engaged in a variety of administrative tasks.

update Following the move to Acorn Lodge, Monday ceased to be dominated by meetings throughout the morning, although another regular meeting, that of the Cosham Continuing Care Group, took place in the afternoon. This was attended by three CPNs, the two social workers and the Continuing Care Specialist with a city-wide brief. Another indication of the growth in activities associated with continuing care developments was the contact which individual team members from the community office had with the residential unit in two of the recorded weeks, regarding the use of an identified respite care bed. Whilst the regular contact club continued to operate on Monday afternoons, it was now the primary responsibility of the OT helper.

Tuesday For some team members, for example the four CPNs, Tuesday during the pre-move period was used mainly to visit clients in their own homes. These visits were punctuated by calls back to their office base to deal with telephone messages and carry out other administrative tasks. On some occasions visits were made jointly, perhaps with another member of the team or, as recorded in one week by a CPN, with a social worker from the local social services area centre.

Cosham Health Centre was used on Tuesdays by a number of staff members. In the mornings the social worker, along with a colleague from the Wessex Unit and a nurse therapist from Vinten House, worked there together as the 'family therapy team'. One CPN generally spent Tuesday afternoons there, seeing clients by appointment for individual counselling sessions. The psychologist also held a regular Tuesday afternoon session at this location, generally seeing clients on an individual basis. During the first recorded week however, she and one of the CPNs attended a study day on supervision, held at the main hospital.

The senior OT recorded a regular Tuesday morning activity at Vinten House, where she was involved in a health education group for current residents. In week 2 she attended a lunchtime briefing meeting to receive management information from the Area Manager for the city.

Other regular Tuesday activities were the two outpatient clinics held in the morning at the Battenburg Avenue Health Centre, undertaken by the associate specialist and the registrar. The consultant psychiatrist's involvement on Tuesdays was generally limited to dealing with correspondence and telephone calls, although in the first recorded week he spent some time interviewing an 'overdose patient' at the local general hospital.

A focal point for many of the team in week 2 was a case presentation by two members of the Cosham team: a CPN and a nurse therapist based at Vinten House. This was a formal presentation to a multidisciplinary group in the main hospital. Many other Cosham team members attended this meeting, which was chaired by the consultant psychiatrist.

update Whilst the Cosham Health Centre continued to be used on Tuesdays by one of the social workers, in his capacity as a member of the family therapy team, it was no longer used for individual counselling sessions either by the CPN or the full-time psychologist who had previously used it. Other changes to be noted were the discontinuation of any formal input by the senior OT into the residential unit and the regular contact established by one CPN with a local GP surgery.

Another important development in the service recorded in the second logging exercise was the setting up of the Sevenoaks Club, a drop-in day care facility operating in a local community centre. Generally, several team members based in the community office visited the club, although it was the OT helper who maintained a regular commitment to spending most of the day there.

Wednesday The range of activities in which the North Lodge staff were involved on Wednesdays was very varied and illustrates many different facets of the service in operation in the period prior to its move to Acorn Lodge. For two CPNs the main focus of the day was on visiting people in their own homes. As usual their activities were interwoven with time spent at North Lodge engaged in informal discussion with colleagues, responding to messages, and dealing with a range of administrative tasks.

A local community centre was the scene of considerable activity on a

Wednesday. During the first part of the morning one CPN ran a weekly relaxation group, and had recently begun to involve the OT helper in these sessions. This was followed by a women's support group, jointly run by another CPN and the senior OT. The latter sometimes used these occasions to see some clients individually, although in week 3 she spent the entire morning at a team briefing workshop run by the personnel officers from both St James' and Coldeast Hospitals. This was also attended by twenty-five other 'team briefers' from these two hospitals.

The clinical psychologist had a regular Wednesday morning commitment seeing individual clients at the Battenberg Avenue Health Centre, in the southern part of the area. This activity was recorded in weeks 2 and 3, although throughout week 1 the psychologist was duty officer, and on the Wednesday in particular her activities were dominated by this commitment. Her morning dealing with correspondence and telephone calls had been interrupted by a request for a home assessment with a view to possible admission. Having gathered together as much information as possible from a number of telephone calls to the GP and other team members, she visited the client at home. She then returned to base to liaise further with team colleagues at both North Lodge and Vinten House, and to keep the GP informed of events.

The social worker's day was less structured than those of some of his colleagues, although his time was also spent both in direct client contact and at 'home base'. One distinctive feature of his activities was contact with various social services colleagues, as exemplified in week 1 when he spent time at the local area centre.

By the second week of logging, monthly 'briefing groups' had been introduced throughout the District. Consequently, a briefing meeting took place at lunchtime on the Wednesday, to communicate information received on the previous day by the senior OT, as team briefer. All the CPNs, the psychologist and the OT helper attended this meeting.

Interwoven with these, broadly speaking, client-related activities, several team members were also involved in a range of discussions concerning future developments in the service. For example, in the second and third recorded weeks, two CPNs, the senior OT and the psychologist spent the early part of the Wednesday afternoon at a meeting which was also attended by two representatives from the local social services area centre and a staff nurse from the District-wide rehabilitation team. This group was involved in the planning and setting up of a day care project for clients requiring continuing care. On one occasion it met at the area centre and on the other at North Lodge. We have already seen from our 'update' to Tuesday that this project had come to fruition by the second period of logging.

The OT helper spent her Wednesday afternoons at Vinten House with any residents wishing to join in a group cookery session. Once again the consultant psychiatrist spent the bulk of his day in work related to the

District Drug Service, although he generally managed to call at North Lodge to deal with correspondence.

update Following the move to Acorn Lodge, Wednesday replaced Monday as the main morning for meetings. The day began with a referrals meeting, chaired by a staff member and regularly attended by a representative from the local social services office. This meeting was followed by the now fortnightly business meeting, which on the part of staff from the residential unit was only attended during weeks 4, 5 and 6 of logging by the Clinical Manager or another single representative.

One important feature of Wednesday mornings which remained unchanged throughout the study period was the weekly relaxation group, followed by a women's support group. However, these were now activities primarily led by the OT helper, who later in the day was also involved in a swimmers' group which had recently been established.

There was an increase between the two logging periods in the time being spent by several team members in attending meetings: in particular meetings either associated with the general development of services for people with longer-term problems or, as in one logging week, related to the management of the newly-established Sevenoaks Club. The latter's management committee was chaired by the senior OT and attended by one CPN and one of the social workers; it also involved representatives from other statutory agencies and voluntary organizations.

At the same time, the diversity of work across the team was illustrated by the other social worker, who recorded time spent during one afternoon on a range of essentially child-focused client-related activities.

Thursday For one of the CPNs and the psychologist, Thursdays during the pre-move period began with attendance at a policy group meeting held at North Lodge. This was also attended by one of the clinical teachers/joint appointees and the Clinical Manager from Vinten House, and in week 1 of logging by the registrar. At what was a regular Thursday morning meeting, a range of policy issues was generally explored. On one occasion there was much discussion regarding the general lack of resources for the development of the service, and on another occasion the role of the Intensive Care Unit was discussed.

After this meeting the CPN, like her colleagues, made some home visits. She then returned to North Lodge to give supervision to a student nurse. The senior OT also visited some clients at home, before making her weekly contact with the Highclere Unit, the residential detoxification unit which forms part of both District and Regional Drug Services, where she ran a relaxation group. The OT helper spent her morning visiting two clients in their own homes.

A regular feature on Thursday afternoons was another contact club. This one was held at a local community centre and known as 'the Grove

Club'. It involved the CPN identified earlier as regularly attending the Monday contact club. Sometimes other CPNs attended, as recorded during one week when a CPN took a client to the club and then spent some time participating in the group activities and talking with one or two of the attenders individually. There was also a regular input by volunteers.

In week 2 the contact club did not meet in its normal way, since it was the day of the annual outing, mainly organized for club members. On this occasion there was a day trip to Henley-on-Thames and Windsor, the party consisting of 21 clients, 10 family members or friends, 2 volunteers, 3 team members (2 CPNs and the senior OT) and a student OT. The day was a long one, and as one staff member recorded:

> *An outing sounds like a nice day out, but involves clearing up vomit, pushing wheelchairs, finding lost people, stopping one chap running off to thumb a lift, stopping some chap using the roadside emergency phone to call an ambulance when not needed, and stopping agoraphobic people panicking on the coach and on the boat trip. Got home at 7.30, utterly shattered.*

Another feature of Thursday afternoons was the relaxation group, which was run by the same CPN as that held on Wednesday mornings, although at a different community centre. As with the other session, the OT helper was taking direct responsibility for the running of the group, but the CPN was present in a supervisory capacity. After the session there was usually an opportunity for informal conversation amongst the group attenders, with time also made available by the CPN to see individuals if necessary.

The psychologist's day was also a mixture of activities, some client-related and others essentially service development work. Over the pre-move logging period she recorded a good deal of time spent drafting policy documents and recording meetings related to the setting up of the day care project referred to earlier. In week 1 she made a home visit on the Thursday afternoon, followed by an appointment with another client at the Cosham Health Centre in the early evening. On another Thursday she spent time at Vinten House with a client. The additional clinical psychologist held her second session at Cosham Health Centre on Thursdays.

The social worker's activities on a Thursday also varied considerably over the pre-move period. In one week much of his morning was spent in court with a client. He then visited another client at Vinten House and spent most of the afternoon engaged in report writing and telephone calls concerning other individual clients. In his other recorded week he spent Thursday morning at Cosham Health Centre, seeing clients individually and (together with a co-worker) meeting a married couple. During the afternoon he spent some time with a client whom he accompanied to Vinten House for a brief visit, dealt with various administrative tasks, and received his regular social work supervision.

On Thursdays the consultant psychiatrist was again primarily involved in work with the drug services. However, he generally made a brief visit to North Lodge to deal with correspondence. On one Thursday he spent time with a client, preparing a court report, which he then discussed with the probation officer concerned. He then went to Vinten House to see a resident and to discuss her situation with both the social worker and some members of the Vinten House staff.

update By the second series of logging weeks, a weekly support group for all team members based in the community office was being held regularly on Thursday mornings. The weekly review of residential clients took place in the afternoon, with some representation from the community team.

Two regular features of Thursday afternoon, the contact club and the relaxation group, both held at local community centres, continued throughout the study period, although changes took place in relation to the staffing input. Regular staff presence at the contact club was maintained on a rota basis, involving either one of three CPNs or the senior OT. The OT helper now had responsibility for the relaxation group, albeit with access to supervision.

Substantially more meetings associated with the planning of future services were recorded throughout the second logging period. For example, one social worker was involved in plans related to the development of sheltered accommodation, whilst the other reported a number of activities in the context of his membership of the executive of MIND and his work with a group for sex offenders. One CPN, who was involved in discussions with a city-wide sports co-ordinator concerning the development of 'Portsmouth Interaction', also regularly attended a carers'/family support group meeting.

Friday In the first period of logging, the CPNs and the social worker were mainly using Fridays to visit clients at home and to deal with a range of administrative tasks at North Lodge. In week 1, one CPN and the social worker, along with a social work colleague from another mental health service patch team, attended an open day held by a community mental health team in London.

The OT regularly spent part of Friday morning at Vinten House, running a 'personal care' group for residents. During one recorded week she attended a meeting with the community worker from the local social services area centre and the staff nurse from the rehabilitation unit, to discuss the use of volunteers for the continuing care day care project, by then named 'the Sevenoaks Club'. Having spent the early part of the afternoon seeing clients at home, she returned to North Lodge to record her activities and complete other administrative tasks, in the company of fellow team members.

The consultant psychiatrist's input varied considerably as between the three recorded Fridays. On one occasion he spent a short time dealing with correspondence, followed by a domiciliary visit. On another Friday he spent the afternoon preparing a court report, which involved him in seeing the client and a relative, then discussing the situation with both the probation officer and the key worker, a nurse therapist from Vinten House. On the Friday of the third recorded week he was on annual leave. Friday was a regular research study day for the psychologist.

update The Sevenoaks Club was a regular feature of Fridays during the second period of logging; it now operated from 12 noon until 4 p.m., with the OT helper once again substantially involved. In addition, there were other continuing care service activities, focused around meetings: for example those involving one of the social workers with the Portsmouth Housing Association concerning the development of sheltered accommodation.

Friday also remained a day of considerable direct client-related work during the second logging period. There were specific examples of joint work recorded by individual team members; for example one CPN acting as the duty officer involved another team member in a joint assessment, which took up most of the morning.

As the foregoing example indicates, the duty system, which had been changed to a daily rota by the time of the second period of logging, impinged considerably on the activities of the team member concerned on some specific occasions. We noted this earlier, with an example from the first logging period. However, the impact of being duty officer varied considerably; it could - and generally did - mean little disturbance to the planned day's activities, but it sometimes brought substantial involvement with a client and extensive negotiations with other professional colleagues. In logging week 6, a meeting to review the duty officer system was attended by several team members from the community office and the Clinical Manager from the residential unit.

Summary This description of the day-by-day work of those team members based initially at North Lodge and subsequently at Acorn Lodge, both confirms and develops the pattern which was evident from the analysis of activities based on location. During the whole period covered by our two logging exercises, almost all of the team's direct contact with clients took place out in the Cosham area, away from base, either in people's own homes or in local community or health centres. At North Lodge or in the community office at Acorn Lodge, much of their time was spent on administrative tasks and on informal team contact.

Whilst home visiting remained an important feature of these staff's activities throughout the period covered by the logging studies, our descriptive account has highlighted an increasing use of non-domestic local settings, particularly in the development of services for continuing care clients. For example, what was being planned as a drop-in day care facility during the first logging exercise had become an integral part of the Cosham service by the time the second period of logging took place. In addition, many of the activities and developing facilities indicated by the first set of logging data continued to operate on a regular basis, relying to a considerable extent on the increasing involvement of the OT helper, who took primary responsibility for a number of activities previously led by the more highly qualified staff. The latter, in their turn, became increasingly involved in activities associated with the planning and development of services.

The logging studies revealed a number of important and substantial changes in the roles and tasks of some team members over time, within an overall context of both maintaining and expanding services. By the second logging period, following the coming together of the whole service at Acorn Lodge, much of the CPNs' and the senior OT's time had come to be spent in negotiating and planning service developments, rather than on direct work with individual clients. Other changes over time, of a different nature, resulted in the loss of certain activities or facilities. For example, the absence of the full-time clinical psychologist and the reduction in the number of hours worked by the senior OT led to a reduction in specialist inputs to the service.

Prior to the move, relatively little time was spent by staff based at North Lodge at the overall team's other accommodation on the main hospital site, Vinten House, except when attending the weekly business meeting. The latter provided an opportunity for the whole team to get together, as did other more individually-focused activities such as joint work as part of the family therapy team. Following the move, the areas of overlap between those team members based in the community office and those based in the new residential unit remained mainly in the area of shared work with individual clients. Whilst most of the 'community team' regularly attended the referral and business meetings, these were only infrequently attended by residentially-based staff, other than the Clinical Manager or Assistant Clinical Manager, and no longer provided an opportunity for regular team contact.

The foregoing account of the community team's activities has indicated a degree of overlap and of sharing tasks within the team as a whole. One example was the work undertaken in the assessment of new referrals to the service, to which the residentially-based staff, with their community focus, made a significant contribution throughout the period studied. This is explored more fully in the next section, through a detailed examination of the work undertaken by those team members based in the residential unit.

Residentially-based staff

Any account of the activities of staff based in the residential unit forming part of the Cosham Mental Health Service, as Vinten House in the pre-move period and when located at Acorn Lodge subsequently, must reflect two interconnecting strands: work undertaken in the residential setting itself and activities in the local community. We first offer a detailed description of the former, by means of 'a typical day and night' in the life of Vinten House during the period of our first logging exercise. This is followed by a description of the activities undertaken further afield by staff based at Vinten at that time, many of which took place on particular days of the week. Then we give an update on the activities of this group of staff following their move to the residential unit within Acorn Lodge. The section concludes with some observations regarding changes over time.

'A typical day and night' It is not easy to convey a sense of a day and night in the life of Vinten House, since no such period was completely typical. Data from the first logging period suggest that the weekends were very different from the weekdays, when there were more comings and goings of Vinten House staff and other team members. Mondays were different from other weekdays because of the regular meetings held in the House. Nevertheless, each day had an underlying pattern, imposed to a large extent by the system of providing twenty-four-hour care on a three-shift system - early duty from 7.30 a.m. to 3 p.m., late duty from 2.30 p.m. to 10 p.m., and night duty from 9.30 p.m. to 8 a.m. - and by the day-to-day habits and routines of the residents themselves.

One starting point to the day was the handover meeting between the night duty therapist and the early duty therapist. Around this time residents were beginning to get up and the therapist coming on duty had an opportunity to greet the residents and to familiarize her/himself with the general atmosphere of the House and the possible needs of each resident.

Throughout the day the duty therapist undertook a wide range of tasks necessary to the day-to-day management of the House. This inevitably involved a good deal of informal contact with residents and with other staff members. The chief characteristic was constant interruption, whether by a resident with a specific request, or by a telephone call from another member of the Cosham team, from a relative of a current resident, or an enquiry from a professional working in the local community. Whatever it might be it had to be dealt with, and tasks such as 'paperwork' were temporarily put aside to be picked up later, when more pressing demands had been satisfied. Sometimes the pace was hectic; at other times little seemed to be happening and there were opportunities for an informal chat with a colleague, or time to sit with residents, who generally occupied the communal sitting room.

The handover from the early to the late shift occurred at 3 p.m. and the late duty therapist then provided cover through the rest of the afternoon and most of the evening. The earlier pattern of activities continued during this period of duty, although by the early evening there were usually increased opportunities to spend time with the residents before they retired to bed. For example, in the second week of logging the duty therapist recorded amongst her activities time spent with an individual resident, before joining a group of residents in the communal sitting room. Later in the evening an ex-resident, who was very distressed, called at the House; time was spent with her, prior to completing the day's report and handing over to the night duty therapist.

There was a further opportunity for informal contact, between the night duty therapist and residents, during the late evening, and some time was spent with individual residents during the night, if for example they were having difficulties sleeping. There was generally also time at night for the completion of routine administrative tasks.

An attempt was made to organize the duty rota in such a way that the duty therapist had additional in-house support during most of the day. This task might be shared between staff members over the course of a day, giving the duty therapist some flexibility in the House, so that s/he could spend time with individual clients, supervise a student nurse, or receive personal supervision.

Occasionally, as in the first logging week, the needs of the particular resident group required further support in the House. One resident was needing continual observation and special nursing care, which meant that another staff member had to be available at all times to share the tasks of providing in-house cover. The decision to provide the additional cover for this resident, enabling her to remain in the House rather than be transferred to the Intensive Care Unit (Brunel Villa), had implications for all staff. Extra in-house support was provided with the help of some experienced student nurses, whose input was recognized as having a learning component; supervision and support were necessarily provided at all times.

For the outsider visiting Vinten House, there were some occasions when there was an atmosphere of calm, whilst at other times there was great activity. To some extent this reflected the characteristics of a normal domestic environment, with ups and downs depending on the activities and moods of the occupants. The atmosphere of home was more evident at the weekends; there were fewer interruptions from outside callers and the residents had the House much more to themselves. They were encouraged to participate in household tasks and activities, and this was an important part of the weekend, when neither the housekeeper nor the nursing assistant worked. As an example, in the third recorded week the early duty therapist on the Saturday started her morning with the regular handover session, then helped prepare breakfast, which she and the residents ate together. Most of the morning was spent with everyone involved in generally tidying and cleaning the House, during which time the nurse therapist could both talk with and listen to the residents. After lunch she spent time in the company of the residents as they relaxed together after their busy morning.

However, it was not always possible to maintain this sort of atmosphere, even at the weekends. For example, on the first Sunday recorded, the early duty therapist spent a considerable part of her duty session making telephone calls and generally liaising with medical staff and other colleagues within the hospital, mainly concerning a new resident who had been admitted the previous night. Nevertheless, the duty therapist found time to offer supervision to a student nurse and to join in cooking and eating lunch with the residents.

From this description it is evident that a substantial amount of time was being spent by all staff based at Vinten House in providing in-house cover and support. In addition to this, they also had some time allocated for work with clients not resident at Vinten House. Formally, five of each individual's ten sessions in a fortnight were allocated for duty in the House, with the remainder being given over to 'community work'. In practice, as we have already indicated, these proportions varied over time. Some work with non-resident clients did take place within the House, but it was those aspects of the staff's work which took place away from Vinten House which were more readily described as 'community work'. During our first logging exercise, some examples of such activities were very similar to those carried out by the North Lodge-based staff group, for example domiciliary visiting, whereas others represented an additional or alternative form of intervention. These activities, which often involved more than one staff member and many of which formed a regular feature or commitment of a particular day of the week, can best be outlined on a day-by-day basis.

Weekly features Mondays, as already indicated, were dominated during the pre-move period by a number of meetings, some of which took place at Vinten House. The pattern of these meetings changed over the first logging period. During week 1 Vinten House had its own business meeting during the late morning; this represented an opportunity to discuss House matters. In the early part of the afternoon the Vinten House staff held their support group, which was followed by the regular Vinten House review meeting. By the second week of logging the Vinten House support group was meeting in the late morning, prior to the newly established business meeting for all members of the Cosham team, which was followed in turn by the Vinten House review.

Several Vinten House staff sought to attend both the business and the review meetings, although there were constraints of time, duty rota and community commitments for each nurse therapist to negotiate. The

Clinical Manager and the two clinical teachers/joint appointees were, however, regular attenders. Whilst these meetings provided a useful opportunity for more contact amongst the wider team, with increased numbers of staff involved there was inevitably some intrusion into the domestic life of the House. This exemplifies the conflicting demands made on Vinten House as a result of its functioning as both an organizational and a service/domestic base.

On Tuesdays, several nurse therapists had regular commitments involving the use of the Cosham Health Centre. One nurse therapist regularly spent her morning at this location, working with the family therapy team, whilst two of her colleagues spent the afternoon there offering joint counselling sessions to couples.

A regular feature of work recorded on Wednesdays was the early evening group for abused women, jointly run by two nurse therapists and held at a local church hall.

A psycho-drama group run by a nurse therapist and a colleague from another team met each Thursday. On the Thursday of the third week of logging, two nurse therapists attended a workshop on co-counselling. Whilst this was a particular training/educational activity, it illustrates the shared commitment of team members to both personal professional development and to the education and training of others. A further example of this commitment is the task of supervising student nurses, which was going on throughout the week.

There were no particular events regularly associated with Fridays. As on other days, some clients were visited at home. There was also an emphasis on providing in-house support, which might possibly include an individual session with a client, supervision of a student nurse, personal supervision, administrative tasks, or informal contact with residents.

This account of Vinten House in terms of its staff's activities has so far largely omitted the input from the Clinical Manager and the two clinical teachers/joint appointees. The latter had important educational roles and made a major contribution to activities within the Nurse Training Unit, whilst remaining in touch with practice through direct work with clients and general involvement in the wider Cosham Mental Health Team. A brief description of one day recorded in the second week of logging by one of the clinical teachers illustrates this range of activities and how it related to the overall work of the Cosham team. This clinical teacher started her day with personal supervision, then taught a group of general nursing students. Later in the morning she was in direct contact with a client. The early part of the afternoon was spent at Vinten House, where she had informal contact with both staff and residents. Then she attended a psycho-drama special interest group with one of the nurse therapists.

An important feature of the Clinical Manager's role is highlighted by her attendance at all the regular Monday meetings. During the remainder of the week her activities were more varied, although many could broadly be described as 'liaison' or 'co-ordination'. For example, the following description of her work as recorded for a Tuesday in the second logging week was broadly typical of all three recorded weeks during the pre-move period.

The Clinical Manager started her day with some informal contact with colleagues and residents at Vinten House, before discussing House policies and practices with a senior tutor from the Nurse Teaching Unit. She then dealt with various administrative tasks, general enquiries and telephone calls at Vinten House, before having a one-to-one session with a client. In the afternoon she attended a team briefing session at Cavendish House with the Manager of the City Mental Health Services. On her return she was involved in a discussion of the needs of one resident with the registrar and one of the clinical teachers. She spent the rest of the afternoon giving support to various staff members and supervising a student nurse. This description also highlights another dimension of the Clinical Manager's role: namely providing in-house support to the duty therapist and, less formally, to other Vinten House-based colleagues.

Update The preceding account of the pattern of daily and weekly activities of staff based at Vinten House during our first logging period has attempted to convey something of the nature and diversity of this particular unit. In addition to offering residential care to a small number of residents in an essentially domestic setting, Vinten House was offering various other forms of help to people living in the Cosham area. Recorded staff activities included individual contact with clients in their own homes, at a local health centre, and at Vinten House, as well as working with groups of clients with similar needs.

Examined by means of data from our second logging exercise, the life of the residential unit by then located within Acorn Lodge appears very similar in many respects to that of Vinten House. There was a broadly similar structure to the day, with three duty therapists providing twenty-four-hour care throughout the week. However, some important changes had taken place: the loss of the two joint appointees who had been specifically attached to Vinten House, the creation of an Assistant Clinical Manager post, and the more recent introduction of support workers, sharing the day-to-day running of the House with the duty therapist.

There appeared to be a high degree of informality in the contacts between all staff and residents, as they shared together in the daily life of the unit. It was also evident from the accounts supplied both by the nurse therapists and the support workers that there was considerable overlap between the tasks undertaken by the latter and by the duty nurse therapist. However, in addition to this overlapping of tasks, there were some clear divisions of responsibility. The duty nurse therapist was in charge of the unit and had administrative and professional responsibilities to carry out. Supervision of medication, handling specific enquiries about a resident's well-being, and contact with other professional colleagues, took up substantial proportions of the duty therapist's time, along with supervising the support workers. These tasks were inevitably interwoven with other activities: more informal contacts with residents and staff, supervision of a student nurse, and some administrative work.

The more routine and regular interactions of domestic life essentially took place between the support workers and residents. For example, the housekeeper was usually involved in the preparation of meals and this frequently provided a time for talking informally with some of the residents, who might join him in this task. Time was also spent sitting with residents, sharing in their conversations, or joining in a game of cards. Whereas previously this in-house support had been provided wherever possible by the nurse therapists, it was now an activity which was being carried out and developed by the support workers. There were several recorded accounts of a support worker accompanying residents to the local shops, to the Sevenoaks Club, or in one case on an appearance at the local court.

In the first logging exercise, the nurse therapists had recorded substantial amounts of time spent in providing general in-house cover. This activity was less prominently mentioned in the second logging exercise, where it was replaced by more specific one-to-one direct contact. This took place within Acorn Lodge, although it was not always clear from the logging accounts whether individual clients were being seen in the residential unit itself or in the interviewing rooms located 'on the community side'. Residential staff's work with non-resident clients was taking place within the new base of the whole service, and represented a substantial contribution to the overall team's community work. It included both initial assessment and ongoing contact; along with home visiting it represented an obvious area of overlap with the work of staff based in the community office. However, the residential staff's apparent preference for using Acorn Lodge to see clients living at home was not shared by most of their fellow team members based in the community office; the latter, as we observed earlier, continued to see most of their clients away from home base.

The important liaison and co-ordination activities associated with the role of the Clinical Manager were again highlighted in the second logging exercise. In the absence of the Assistant Clinical Manager, who was on sick leave for two of the second three recorded weeks, the Clinical Manager spent as much time within the residential unit as on activities further afield. Her regular attendance at the referral and business meetings was again underlined, and had become increasingly important in maintaining links between the two arms of the service.

Thus whilst continuing to provide residential care for a small number of residents in an essentially domestic setting, now located within the community served, the residentially-based staff became increasingly involved in working with clients living in their own homes. These clients were most likely to be invited to attend Acorn Lodge; to a lesser extent they were visited at home. There was no recorded use of other locally-based health or community centres by residentially-based staff during the second logging period. However, their community-orientated activities closely connected with much of the work undertaken by those team members based in the community office, primarily in the area of assessing new referrals. This illustrates how the two parts of the overall service fitted together to provide a variety of help to meet an equally wide range of personal need.

Summary

In this chapter we have examined the activities of members of the Cosham team based at North Lodge and their colleagues based at Vinten House during the months preceding the overall team's proposed move from the St James' Hospital site into the community - the pre-move period. We have compared the main features evident then with the subsequent situation when the whole team was operating from its new community base, Acorn Lodge, and identified any significant changes over time, as the service developed. To do this we have drawn upon data from two series of three logging weeks, six weeks in all, during which team members themselves recorded their work activities. We have analyzed and presented this data, first from the perspective of where staff spent their time and then in terms of their day-by-day activities. The second approach served to complement and extend the understanding of the operation of the service provided by the first.

North Lodge provided an organizational and administrative base for the whole Cosham team, prior to the move of at first only one part of that team to Acorn Lodge. However, it served much more clearly as such a base for the staff actually located there. They went out from and returned to North Lodge and carried out most of their service-providing activities in people's homes and/or in community and health centres in the Cosham area. To a lesser extent, Vinten House was also an organizational/administrative base, but only for the staff mainly working there, who by virtue of the House being a residential facility did much of their direct client-related work there too.

To look in greater detail at staff's more specific activities, we found it necessary to acknowledge the twenty-four-hour cycle at the residential unit as a fundamental structure, around which additional staff activities on particular days, and especially client-related work away from the unit, become more or less possible. The pattern of activities of staff based initially at North Lodge and then in the community office fell more neatly into a 'typical week' (of five days), although an important day-to-day administrative structure pertained there.

A broadly similar pattern of activities was evident from both logging studies, suggesting considerable continuity over time. Even when the whole team was based in the same building, Acorn Lodge, individuals continued mainly to operate either from the community office or from the residential unit, whichever was their respective home base. However, there was some indication of a more widely-shared use of interviewing facilities at Acorn Lodge.

It was clear from the first logging exercise that much of the overall service was already being provided in the local community, in a number of different locations, and that this was how and where the overlapping activities of staff based at North Lodge or at Vinten House were coming together to provide a broad range of community orientated services. The second phase of logging indicated that areas of overlapping activity between the two arms of the service, now united on one site, remained focused around work with individual clients, although the range of community locations used - beyond Acorn Lodge itself - was reduced. Local health centres appeared to be used much less by all team members. Staff based in the new residential unit seemed more inclined to use facilities at Acorn Lodge to see clients from the community than did their colleagues based in the community office. The latter also tended to make more use of community centre locations, reflecting their growing involvement in work with continuing care clients.

The increased involvement of residentially-based staff in one-to-one client contact during the second logging period, reflects to a large extent the contribution made by the introduction of support workers into the residential unit. This released time for additional community work, primarily involving the assessment of newly-referred clients. Similarly, the extensive use of the OT helper in maintaining a number of community-based activities, albeit with supervision, made it possible for some members of the community team to devote more time to a range of service-development activities, particularly in the field of continuing care.

The first logging exercise clearly revealed the multi-faceted nature of the service; this was further underlined by the second phase of recording. Together, the data present a diverse picture of activities within the overall developing service. The complex interplay between the different aspects of the service in the context of providing residential care, developing services for continuing care clients, assessing new referrals, and sustaining a range of client interventions, was revealed in a number of ways. The 'non-traditional' community role of those based in the residential unit was clearly demonstrated, highlighting an important area of overlap and flexibility within the total service. This had continued and extended alongside a greater involvement of non-professionally qualified support workers. There had been a move towards increased diversification of the service as such, accompanied by greater diversity of work within the team, for example in the setting up of a specialist group of team members primarily committed to working in the continuing care arena. In the next chapter we examine the development of services for those people with mental health problems requiring continuing care: a context in which local collaborative working assumes particular importance.

3 Collaborative activities

Introduction

This chapter looks in more detail at one particular aspect of the development of the Cosham Mental Health Service, namely the relationships and collaborative links established with other local agencies and networks during its transition from a hospital to a community base. It will become evident how, in keeping with our overall approach to this study, we have drawn together a range of data from various sources to provide a picture of this area of work.

The main focus of the first part of this chapter is an examination of the mental health work undertaken with individuals by staff of the local area centre of Hampshire Social Services Department, which is situated in Cosham, some 400 yards from Acorn Lodge. To gain some understanding of this, we sought to identify the possible areas of overlap between the two agencies during the period when the 'community' team within the overall Cosham Mental Health Service was moving to its new local base. The first section of the chapter concludes with a discussion of the two agencies' attempts to manage areas of overlap, primarily in relation to the processing of new referrals to the Cosham Mental Health Service.

The second part of the chapter explores particular aspects of collaborative activity related to the development of services for continuing care clients. A joint initiative in the setting up of a drop-in centre for people with longer-term mental health problems is described, along with other developments in this area of work. The views of some users of these services conclude the chapter.

Links with the local social services area centre

Our account of the background and early development of community mental health services in Cosham (Chapter 1) offered some evidence of collaborative activities between the two statutory agencies primarily concerned. For example, there were regular monthly meetings between social workers from the local area centre and the consultant psychiatrist and the CPNs working in the locality. These monthly meetings were initially set up to provide a forum for the exchange of information concerning clients known to both services and for clarifying areas of joint work. When the Cosham Mental Health Service was established, the group broadened its membership to include other team members, more specifically the clinical psychologist, the senior OT, and the Clinical Manager from the residential unit. At the same time other social workers from the area centre were also encouraged to attend the meetings. This initiative was taken by local social services staff, essentially to promote their own work in the mental health field.

Whilst the main focus of these joint meetings continued to be on work concerning individual clients, there was a broadening of the topics discussed to include recent developments by the community mental health team and its plans for moving from the hospital into a local base. This opportunity for the exchange of information became increasingly important when, at the beginning of January 1988, changes in the overall management of mental health services city-wide led to the discontinuation of the Cosham Liaison Group.

During the first year of our study we adopted several approaches to identifying both the amount of mental health work undertaken by local social services staff and the extent of contact between the two agencies. Staff of the area centre, wishing to raise the profile of mental health work amongst colleagues there, were happy to help us in these tasks.

Mental health work within the social services area centre

A short questionnaire, designed to elicit information about the staff's own estimation of their mental health work and contact with NHS mental health personnel, was distributed to all five teams within the area centre in May 1988. Of the five, three were described as 'generic', one as a 'community resource team', and another as the 'home care team'. The latter, directly responsible to their Area Manager, comprised three home care organizers, two qualified OTs and an OT assistant. The community resource team, managed by the Deputy Area Manager, consisted of a day care officer, a family placement officer (fostering), two community workers, a voluntary services co-ordinator and a home economist. The three generic teams, each managed by an Assistant Area Manager, had minor variations in team composition: team one had five qualified social workers, an adult placement officer and a social services officer; team two had five qualified social workers, of whom two were Approved Social Workers (ASWs), a social services officer, a social work assistant and a family aide; team three had six qualified social workers, one an ASW, and a social work assistant.

Summary of findings Twenty-three out of a possible thirty-nine questionnaires were completed, which represented an overall response rate of 60 per cent. Of the twenty-three respondents, fourteen out of a possible sixteen were qualified social workers from the three generic teams. This higher response rate possibly reflected the more direct relevance of the questionnaire to these team members' current workloads and interests. Questionnaires were also completed by two Assistant Area Managers, the adult placement officer, four members of the community resource team (day care officer, family placement officer, the voluntary services co-ordinator and a community worker), and two members of the home care team (the senior OT and the home care organizer).

Of the twenty-three respondents, nine reported some contact with a Cosham Mental Health Team member during the previous month. This included a group of five social workers, three of whom cited the regular monthly liaison meeting. In addition to this contact, one had had some discussion with the consultant psychiatrist and another had met with members of the residential unit whilst visiting a client. The two other social worker respondents recorded contact with a CPN; one had undertaken a piece of joint work and the other had had some discussion of a case whilst dealing with a duty call. One Assistant Area Manager recorded having chaired the liaison meeting and also having some informal contact with the social worker based in the Cosham Mental Health Team. The adult placement officer had both had discussions and undertaken a joint visit with a CPN, and the voluntary services co-ordinator had had discussions with the clinical psychologist and two CPNs concerning the use of volunteers. One OT also recorded her attendance at the liaison meeting, which she had specifically used to establish contact with the Cosham Mental Health Team's OT.

With the exception of one respondent who felt that all of her/his work had a mental health component, the proportion of overall workload estimated in this way ranged from 0-30 per cent. Table 3.1 shows that slightly more than half of the respondents (13) recorded 5 per cent or less, including six reporting no work of this kind. Eight respondents reported anything between 6 and 30 per cent. The main activities identified within this estimated workload included direct work with clients in their own homes and liaison with the mental health services. Two respondents referred specifically to their ASW activities.

Table 3.1
Percentage of overall workload estimated as 'mental health work'

Estimated percentage	Number of respondents
0%	6
1-5%	7
6-10%	2
11-15%	1
16-20%	2
21-25%	1
26-30%	2
'all'	1
not known	1
Total	23

In response to a question asking whether the amount of mental health work personally undertaken currently was either 'too little', 'about right' or 'too much', seventeen respondents, including ten social workers, felt that the current proportion of their time spent on mental health work was 'about right'. Of the three social workers who felt that they carried out too little such work, two shared a similar view concerning their own lack of training or limited experience. For example, one commented:

Unable to obtain a place on the mental health/ASW course and therefore feel hesitant regarding taking on much mental health work without training or practical knowledge. I need to make a conscious decision to reduce other areas of work to make room for mental health work. This is gradually changing now, but the general expectation in the past was that mental health work should go only to the ASWs in the office.

Another of this group of three respondents expressed some uncertainty regarding her/his role in relation to the members of the Cosham Mental Health Team:

Our role in relation to the CPN service is not always very clearly defined. However, it is an area of work which I am interested in.

One social worker felt that (s)he had too much mental health work. (S)he also held the view that lack of training created uncertainty about such work. However, the liaison meeting was seen as useful:

... in helping social workers to offer an effective service and to enable the community mental health team and the Area social workers to come together. It also offers support and reduces the feelings of working alone.

Of the two Assistant Area Managers who completed the questionnaire, both felt that they undertook too little mental health work. One commented on the Area's commitment to promoting work with clients with mental health problems, and his efforts to encourage this shift. The other felt that there were too few opportunities to gain sufficient experience in mental health work to become sufficiently familiar with both the needs of the client group and the resources available.

Overall, both contact with members of the Cosham Mental Health Team and the amount of work perceived as having a mental health component were very limited, and were mainly focused around a small group of qualified social workers (including three ASWs). The majority of respondents felt that the proportion of mental health work which they personally carried out was 'about right', although both those respondents who wanted more and those who wanted less work of this kind expressed the need for more training and experience in this specialist area.

These findings raise a number of issues pertinent to developing collaborative links between these two agencies. On the part of some area-based social workers there was an interest in pursuing work in the mental health field and developing collaborative activities with the Cosham Mental Health Team. However, with competing demands from client groups given higher priority and limited opportunities for staff development in this field, such activities rested with a small and relatively restricted group of individuals.

In asking individual practitioners to assess the extent to which their work could be said to have a mental health component, we were aware of a likely under-estimation of the incidence of mental health problems, which may well have been present in a significant number of cases (Fisher, Newton and Sainsbury, 1984; Huxley and Fitzpatrick, 1984). This was an area further pursued through an examination of mental health referrals made to the area centre over a ten-month period.

Monitoring mental health referrals to the area centre

As a means of assessing the impact of the decentralizing Cosham Mental Health Service on the local social services area centre's mental health work, a system of monitoring mental health referrals to the area centre was established. Staff of Hampshire Social Services Department, both from the area centre in Cosham and at county headquarters in Winchester, were actively involved in this task. Using statistical material routinely collected via the department's computerized client information system, it was possible to identify all referral incidents coded as having the presenting problem 'mental disorder', and those which at the time of an allocation decision were given the client group code 'mentally ill'. However, as indicated at the end of the preceding sub-section, we were aware of a possible under-reporting of the incidence of mental health problems, which may well have been present in a number of cases where the work done was, for example, coded via 'family', 'child(ren) in care' etc., rather than 'mentally ill'.

In order to gain a more detailed and accurate picture of the mental health work undertaken by area-based social workers in Cosham, additional information was collected at the initial assessment stage, when the referral form was passed to the team manager for an allocation decision. At this point the question: 'Is there a mental health component to this case?', was posed in all cases where the work done was coded using a client group code other than 'mentally ill'. If the answer was an affirmative one at this stage, or at the subsequent first review stage, then this was recorded using a series of secondary codes. In an attempt to achieve some consistency in response to the question posed, it was the task of the relevant team manager rather than each individual social worker to record a response. This task fell primarily to the three Assistant Area Managers involved with the duty system.

Thus an overall estimation of recorded mental health work in the area centre was made by drawing upon three related sets of data: (i) referral incidents where the client's presenting problem was recorded as 'mental disorder'; (ii) referral incidents where the client's problem was subsequently coded 'mentally ill'; (iii) any other referral incidents where the client's problem was considered to have a mental health component at the time of initial assessment or first review. Comparable information was extracted from the computerized client information system concerning all of these referral incidents: month of referral, method and source of referral, presenting problem, and referrer's request. There was some overlap between the three sets of data, for example in the situation where a referral with the recorded presenting problem 'mental disorder' was subsequently given the client group code 'mentally ill', or was categorized as having a 'mental health component' in addition to other primary dimensions. In such cases information was included only once in respect of the relevant referral incident.

Data were collected over a ten-month period, during which the 'community' part of the Cosham Mental Health Team moved to its local base. It had been intended to collect data over a longer period, but with a major redesign and reorganization of Hampshire SSD's Client Information System county-wide, early in 1989, this monitoring exercise came to an abrupt conclusion. As a consequence, information covering the remainder of 1989, when the total move of the Cosham service was effected, is not available.

Summary of findings Tables 3.2, 3.3 and 3.4 present basic data for the ten-month period to the end of February 1989. Referrals made over this period are examined by month, source and method of referral.

A total of 143 incidents of referral to the area centre, either with the presenting problem coded as 'mental disorder', or given the client group code 'mentally ill', or categorized as having a 'mental health component', were recorded between May 1988 and February 1989 inclusive. Whilst there was some month-to-month fluctuation, with the lowest number of referrals recorded in July (10) and the highest number in November (21), there was no noticeable overall increase or decrease in the referral rate over time. It should be recalled that part of the Cosham Mental Health Service moved to its community base midway through this period (October), although the residential facility remained on the hospital site until several months later. This information is shown in Table 3.2.

Table 3.2
Month of referral to area centre, May 1988/February 1989

May	June	July	Aug	Sept	Oct	Nov	Dec	Jan	Feb	Total
14	19	10	11	15	17	21	13	12	11	143

Table 3.3
Source of referral to area centre

Self	38
Intra-departmental	29
Relative/friend	27
Hospital (inpatient)	11
Primary health care team	10
Hospital (outpatient)	6
Police	6
Housing department	5
Voluntary organization	4
Other local authority	3
Education dept/school	2
School psychologist	1
DHSS	1
Total	143

The largest single coded source of referral (38) was 'self'. Table 3.3 shows this, along with the pattern of other referral sources during this period. 'Intra-departmental' referrals (29) made up the second largest group, closely followed by an almost equally large group of referrals from relatives or friends (27). Together, self and relative/friend referrals made up 45 per cent of the overall total. The considerably smaller number of referrals from primary health care teams (10) is worth noting, given that referrals from this source are, after self-referral, the most common category of referral to social services area centres across Hampshire (Hants SSD, 1986).

Table 3.4 shows that by far the largest number of referrals were made by telephone (95). Office calls (23) and letters (22) accounted for most of the other ways of making contact.

Table 3.4
Method of referral to area centre

Telephone	95
Office call	23
Letter	22
Meeting	1
Other	2
Total	143

Tables 3.5 and 3.6 indicate the nature of presenting problems and referrers' requests. Table 3.5 shows that approximately two-thirds (98) of the referral incidents had the recorded presenting problem 'mental disorder'. Of the remainder, a substantial number had recorded presenting problems which indicated some practical difficulty: mainly concerning accommodation (8) and financial matters (8). Self-referrals were highly represented among incidents where the recorded presenting problems were associated with practical difficulties, accounting for all but one of the accommodation problems and three relating to financial matters.

Table 3.5
Presenting problem

Mental disorder	98
Accommodation	8
Financial matters	8
Physical disability	7
Unable to cope	5
Illness	4
Person at risk	3
Emotionally disturbed	1
Social relnship difficulties	1
Homelessness	1
Behaviour difficulties	1
Socially isolated	1
Other	5
Total	143

Table 3.6 shows that over half of the requests made by referrers were either for information/advice/advocacy (45) or for social work investigation/assessment (38). Approximately half of the referrers' requests made to area centres across the county also fall within these two categories (Hants SSD, 1986).

Half of the self-referrals in our sample group involved seeking information and advice (19), whereas half of the relatives referring were requesting either social work intervention/treatment (9) or substitute family care (5). Requests from intra-departmental sources were more widely spread between these three categories: information/advice (9), social work intervention (10), and substitute family care (6).

Table 3.6
Referrer's request

Information/advice/advocacy	45
Social work investigation/assessment	38
Social work intervention/treatment	16
Residential/substitute family care	13
Day care	6
Admission to psychiatric hospital	5
OT assessment	4
Convalescence/aftercare	4
Registration as handicapped	3
Psychiatric regrading	2
Domiciliary support	2
Other	5
Total	143

A number of points can be made on the basis of this summary of findings. Firstly, it is evident that over the period monitored, which included the partial move of the Cosham Mental Health Team to its community base, there was no indication of any change in the extent to which mental health work was undertaken by staff of the local social services area centre. Secondly, almost half of the referrals to the area centre which had a mental health component were made by the person concerned her/himself or by a relative/friend, and a significant number of referrals, particularly among this sub-group, involved practical problems or requests for practical resources.

Few of the referrals to the area centre of people with mental health problems were made by GPs, although the latter may have encouraged a number of the clients referring themselves for social services help to do so. As we shall see in Chapter 4, GPs were overwhelmingly the main source of referrals to the Cosham Mental Health Team over a twelve-month period which included the ten months during which information about referrals to the area centre was collated. There was very little evidence of clients themselves actively seeking help from the specialist mental health service on their own initiative.

A number of questions therefore arise about possible areas of overlap between the two local services. For example, were some of the people with mental health problems who sought help from social services, particularly practical help, also in touch with the local mental health service? The data summarized here suggest a need for a more broadly-based investigation of how help with a mental health problem or a related practical problem was initially sought and how, where appropriate, direct contact with the mental health team was established. Further exploration of these issues is the main focus of Chapter 4.

At the beginning of 1989, aware of some overlap between their work and that of social services staff at the local area centre, the Cosham Mental Health Team invited an area centre representative to their weekly referral/allocation meeting. This link was formalized three months later when the Cosham team reviewed its referral procedure. These regular joint discussions of new referrals led to increased co-operation between the two agencies and shared acknowledgement of the need for both services to be more consistent in their recording of areas of overlap, particularly in working with individual clients. A more systematic process of cross-checking new referrals made to the Cosham Mental Health Service with records held by local social services colleagues was subsequently introduced. This procedure in turn facilitated more informed discussion at referral meetings of which might be the most appropriate lead agency. In a small number of situations area centre staff took the initiative in pursuing contact with both the referrer - generally the GP - and the person referred.

The development of more formalized links between local social services staff and the Cosham Mental Health Team in responding to new referrals made to the latter, would suggest a likely increase in the opportunities for joint working and shared learning, and for promoting mental health work within the social services setting. In the next section we focus upon another aspect of collaborative activity between the Cosham Mental Health Service and other local agencies, including once again the local area centre of Hampshire Social Services Department: namely that taking place in the context of developing services for continuing care clients.

Developing continuing care services

Introducing their collection of papers on services for 'the continuing care client', Lavender and Holloway (1988) address the conceptual and practical minefield involved, and suggest that the people concerned are best understood as those needing help over an extended period and commonly experiencing accommodation, financial, and other difficulties related to their mental health problems. It is this feature, rather than particular diagnostic categories, which gives rise to the need for a different response to that required in 'acute' or 'short-term' situations.

In this text so far, we have noted at appropriate points the impact of the concern of the Cosham service to give increased priority to the needs of people with longer-term mental health problems. As one team member put it:

> *Continuing care clients have really been left by the wayside; partly because of the demands of the acute work coming in, but also because everyone thought that it was someone else's responsibility. And it's only now that we're really communicating with all the other agencies and saying 'let's work together': ... joint work, particularly with social services.*

Developing closer collaborative links with other agencies, and in particular with the local social services area centre, became an increasingly important feature of the decentralizing Cosham Mental Health Service during the period of our study. In this section we focus on two specific and related aspects of this collaborative activity: one centres around a particular joint initiative in developing services for people with longer-term mental health problems; the other concerns the setting up of the Cosham Continuing Care Group.

The Sevenoaks Club

In Chapter 1, in recounting the early development of the Cosham service, we described the setting up of a continuing care working party, which evolved a brief to work together in the planning and development of some form of day care provision in the local community. Over the first nine months of 1988, members of the Cosham Mental Health Team and staff from the local social services area centre, in conjunction with the National Schizophrenia Fellowship (NSF), worked together in the setting up of an informal drop-in centre, later to become known as 'the Sevenoaks Club'.

Once a location had been identified, the planning group began to discuss more specific issues concerning the type of facility to be set up. At this stage the mental health team's OT and a CPN, both already involved in work with continuing care clients through the two existing contact clubs, became more fully involved in this venture. There was a generally shared view, strongly articulated by the NSF's Development Officer, that this day care facility would be for people with longer-term mental health problems who were lonely, isolated, and possibly unemployed. Whilst all members of the group wanted to establish a relatively informal social setting, various views were expressed about the degree of structured activity that should be incorporated into the day. Agreement was eventually reached to set up an informal drop-in centre with relatively few formal, structured activities. It was acknowledged, however, that club members might wish to organize more structured activities; in such circumstances the club's co-ordinator/project worker would play an important part in enabling this to happen.

The ways in which the professional workers might work together with both volunteers and users in the development of the club represented another major aspect of the group's discussions throughout this period. In particular, the extent to which the professional workers should have direct involvement in the club's activities was given careful consideration. Eventually it was agreed that, whilst the professional workers would provide a regular rota of cover, the day-to-day responsibility for running the club would rest with the paid co-ordinator. In setting out a job description for this latter post, emphasis was given to the role of the co-ordinator in involving users of the service - to be called 'members' - as much as possible in the running of the club, in conjunction with volunteers and local statutory and voluntary agencies.

The Sevenoaks Club formally opened in October 1988, operating from a local community centre on two days each week. It was funded jointly by the three agencies to which we have already referred, along with a contribution from the local MIND group and other community groups. A paid non-professionally qualified co-ordinator was provided by the mental health service, in the form of a nursing assistant seconded from a MIND day centre based in another part of the city. Some regular professional input came from staff based at the social services area centre and members of the Cosham Mental Health Team.

There were several features associated with this particular venture which seem to have encouraged its relatively swift implementation as a joint initiative. The mental health team's keenness to develop some local facilities for people with longer-term mental health problems, coincided with the interest of area centre staff in developing their mental health work by building stronger community links in a particular locality: one which had been identified as a deprived area, generally lacking in community resources. These enthusiasms also overlapped with the interest of the NSF, who were equally keen to develop local services in conjunction with other agencies.

Furthermore, all three key workers involved in getting this project off the ground had a community development brief as part of their particular posts. Within the area centre this activity was seen as one part of the community worker's brief to develop a range of activities based on this particular community centre. As we have already noted, the Cosham Mental Health Team's clinical psychologist had, at the time of her appointment in the previous year, been given the task of identifying the needs of continuing care clients, with a view to developing services for them. Direct access to managers at a local level with some degree of control over the allocation of resources for local initiatives, both within the mental health service and the area centre, also appears to have been important in getting the facility up and running in the space of a few months.

Many of the issues discussed during the planning stage of the project were worked out in practice during the course of its first year. For all those concerned with the setting up and running of this informal drop-in centre, this was to a large extent a new experience, and one from which many lessons were learned. Members of the Cosham team involved in the venture found that many of their more traditional ways of working directly with clients were being challenged, and that they were having to find ways of extending and developing their skills in working with others, be they other professionals, volunteers or people in the local community. For example, one team member, who had initially joined the project prepared to set up and run a number of structured groups, found herself involved in the recruitment and initial training of volunteers. She later took an active part in the overall management of the club.

For some members of the Cosham Mental Health Team, being involved in this project prompted a growing concern over the relative balance between direct client contact work and service development activities. As one team member explained:

> *I do find it tremendously stimulating being involved in developments ... but as a service is it right that a clinician - a nurse, an OT or whatever - should abandon their clinical work to take on this work. There are different views about this. Is it a personal choice or is it what the service needs, and who makes that choice?*

Increasing involvement in managing the venture and in promoting user involvement became another important aspect of the professionals' contribution to the development of this club. When it was first set up as a joint Health Authority, Social Services Department and NSF project, the planning/steering committee moved into the more formal position of being its management committee, operating under the charitable status of the NSF. During the following year, the committee spent a considerable amount of time drawing up a club constitution and operational policy. It also formally agreed a club philosophy statement, as follows:

> To establish a welcoming, informal environment for people who have had or are currently experiencing mental health difficulties, and to provide the opportunities for companionship, confidence-building and community integration within this relaxed social setting, where members' needs are paramount.

Consistent with the desire to promote the involvement of both club members and the local community, the committee also widened its membership to include elected representatives from the club's membership and the volunteers. Its approach was one of 'working together' rather than of 'outright autonomy', and the committee moved from being a reflection of an essentially professionally-led project to one with a high degree of non-professional involvement. For example, a local community representative and a volunteer took over the posts of chairperson and treasurer, both previously held by Cosham Mental Health Team members.

This gradual reduction - but not withdrawal - of professional input, was mirrored in the day-to-day running of the club. Whilst several members of the Cosham team continued to maintain some regular contact with club members, volunteers and the co-ordinator, day-to-day professional back-up passed to the duty officer based at Acorn Lodge. Furthermore, the six volunteers, working closely with both the co-ordinator and the OT helper, came to provide regular and consistent help in the club, with particular roles in welcoming members on arrival and helping in the preparation of lunch and other refreshments.

In outlining the setting up and early development of this joint initiative, we have highlighted a number of key issues contributing to its early success and its subsequent plans for expansion. The impact on professional practice and the ways in which team members developed new patterns of working have also been explored. Lessons were learned about the setting up of such projects, including the likely pitfalls. Whilst working together with a number of local agencies and networks was a relatively new venture for the Cosham team, the establishment of the Sevenoaks Club represented an important step forward in collaborative working. It also played a part in stimulating interest in working with people with longer-term mental health problems and to some extent encouraged the setting up of the Cosham Continuing Care Group. It is to this more broadly-focused development within the Cosham service that we now turn our attention.

The Cosham Continuing Care Group

Whilst the need to develop services for continuing care clients in the Cosham area was 'on the agenda' from early on in the setting up of the locally-based service, identifying particular team members with a specific brief to work in this field was not seriously addressed until the end of 1988. Shortly after the first stage of the move away from the main hospital site had been accomplished, two workshops were held to give the team an opportunity to share their views about the nature of work with continuing care clients, and their concerns and uncertainties about the impact of forming a specialist group within the overall team. These workshops, facilitated by the Continuing Care Specialist, were attended by the City Manager, most members of 'the community team', and one representative from the residential unit.

In January 1989, the Cosham Continuing Care Group ('the triple-c-g': CCCG) was established. Its members included two CPNs on a full-time basis, along with some involvement from both the senior OT and the clinical psychologist, and the team's two social workers. One nurse therapist from the residential unit also joined the group in a liaison role.

At its first meeting the CCCG discussed and agreed its overall aim thus:

> To identify the needs of people with long-term mental health

problems within the Cosham patch and develop a flexible comprehensive, network of services for this population.

During the period when the CCCG was being formed, the Continuing Care Specialist played an important developmental role by encouraging the group to draw up a shared philosophy and operational policy. There was also much discussion about the types of skills needed to work in this field and how they might be acquired. A paper written at the time by the Continuing Care Specialist identified five main areas of activity: clinical responsibilities, liaison/co-ordination, development of services, education, and research and evaluation. The role of a member of the Cosham Continuing Care Group was also outlined:

> To work as a member of a specialist team in continuing care within the Cosham patch team; to liaise with continuing care teams across the city; to act as the key worker/case co-ordinator for a specified client group; to co-work with colleagues as appropriate; to identify the needs of the client group and their families and participate in the development of services to meet those needs.

Once a group of team members, some of whom would be working exclusively with continuing care clients, had been identified, discussions within this group and at the wider team business meeting focused around how the team as a whole was to manage priorities within the service and its overall workload. In order to develop their work in this relatively under-resourced area, members of the CCCG had to divert their activities away from other areas, for example the assessment of new referrals. As we indicated in Chapter 3, this had a substantial impact on all team members.

Furthermore, as the CCCG became more involved in its developmental and co-ordinating activities, there was increased concern within the group over the relative balance between these activities and those related to direct work with clients. In addition, some workers who were already substantially committed to regular contact with some well-established facilities for continuing care clients, for example the contact clubs and the recently-opened Sevenoaks Club, were keen that these should not be left unsupported as new initiatives demanded attention.

An inter-related issue concerning boundary negotiation, specifically the group's relationship with city-wide developments, was also a focus of attention at the time. During the summer months of 1989 the CCCG met with the Southsea Continuing Care Team to consider how their activities in planning developments both at a patch level and in conjunction with other groups on a city-wide basis could be better co-ordinated. Whilst there was some acknowledgement of the need for a two-tier approach, there were some uncertainties on the part of the CCCG about the nature of its relationships with the overall Cosham team and with the city-wide service.

Given these concerns and some changes in the CCCG's membership, a review of the group's activities was formally undertaken in the autumn of 1989. This review, facilitated by the Continuing Care Specialist, was attended by three CPNs (one newly-appointed to the Cosham service), one social worker, the senior OT, and the Clinical Manager with responsibility for the residential unit. Each team member identified the various activities and developments with which they were involved, and in reviewing these the group was encouraged by its range of achievements. The contact clubs, the women's support group, and the Sevenoaks Club continued to provide a core of facilities in the Cosham area, along with a new resource: the use of a bed in the residential unit at Acorn Lodge for respite care. This latter development was seen as important as it involved more than one part of the overall local Cosham service. Further afield, the group was actively involved in a number of city-wide initiatives; for example in developing accommodation in conjunction with local housing associations. This pattern of activities was revealed in the logging studies, reported in Chapter 2.

Reviewing these developments enabled the group to identify areas of achievement as well as areas for future activity. There was general agreement that it was important to establish an operational policy, which would be helpful in clarifying the boundaries of the CCCG in relation to the overall Cosham team and to city-wide services for continuing care clients. As part of this process, the CCCG also found itself reviewing some aspects of professional practice. One important feature of the group's work with individual clients was the growing amount of co-working being carried out. For example, the senior OT was increasingly using her professional skills in working with others in both joint assessments and in an advisory or consultative role. Another team member had become interested in developing specialist skills for working with clients who were isolated and not easily engaged. This interest, coupled with his commitment to education and training, also gave him the opportunity to encourage students' interest and involvement in continuing care work, thereby promoting the needs of continuing care clients on the educational agenda.

Liaison and co-ordination activities formed another significant area of work for the CCCG. For example, one CPN was working with the 'depot' clinic nurse in the setting up of a monitoring system for clients at risk. Whilst this initiative was still in its early stages, it involved the CPN in a considerable amount of liaison and co-ordination within the Cosham service and across the city. In various ways each member of the group had become involved in the development of new services and facilities, both at a local level and city-wide. Some initiatives have already been mentioned; these included the development of a sheltered accommodation scheme, the setting up of a sports initiative across the city, and a planned expansion of the Sevenoaks Club.

This brief review of the CCCG's activities during its first nine months of life illustrates the key areas of the Cosham team's work which were associated with the development of services for people with longer-term mental health problems. Of these, clinical responsibilities, liaison/co-ordination, service development, and education have been specifically highlighted, whilst the group's participation in a review of its developments demonstrates its active involvement in self-evaluation.

In this chapter so far we have described an example of local collaborative activity between health and social services staff, which brought about the development and joint running of a drop-in day facility in the Cosham area. We have indicated how this particular initiative, along with other factors such as the facilitative role played by the Continuing Care Specialist, contributed to the overall Cosham team's commitment to the setting up of a Cosham Continuing Care Group. The establishment of this group led, in its turn, to further service developments for continuing care clients, some of which have been outlined briefly. The impact of these developments on professional practice has also been explored: existing skills in direct client work were adapted and extended, and new ones, often involving work with other agencies and local networks, were acquired. We now turn our attention to the impact of these developments on the lives of the users of the services concerned.

Users' views

Together, the two well-established contact clubs and the more recently opened Sevenoaks Club came to form what could be considered the 'backbone' of services for continuing care clients in the Cosham area, providing both opportunities for regular social contact, and continuing access to the service and its staff in a relatively informal way. As outlined earlier, the Sevenoaks Club was set up as an informal drop-in facility, where the active involvement of club members and the local community has been encouraged. The contact clubs were seen as more structured than the Sevenoaks Club, and were described by members of the CCCG as:

> *having a basic but flexible routine with a superimposed therapeutic activity.*

All the contact club attenders were known to the service, being either past or present clients. In a few situations a relative accompanied the 'patient'. Both contact clubs operated a follow-up system for people who were absent for an unknown reason, and both had the regular presence of volunteers and a staff member from the Cosham team. At one club the OT helper made a regular input, whilst at the other, one member of the CCCG attended each week on a rota basis.

Interview method An appropriate way of exploring the views and experiences of users of services for continuing care clients seemed to be to take a sample of the people attending either of the two contact clubs or the Sevenoaks Club. We wanted to explore the nature and range of their experiences, feelings and needs, rather than to measure the extent to which the services were used. To do this we identified a number of key issues or topics, drawing on both documentary sources and interviews with the people who had been most intimately involved in developing these services. These issues provided a framework within which users' views could be explored in a flexible but systematic way. Whilst each interview would vary in its emphases, comparable information and users' views on this range of common topics could be collected. The accessibility and acceptability of the services, opportunities for individual choice, and the flexible use of these facilities in conjunction with each other and with other parts of the service, were all seen as key areas for investigation, along with the felt impact of these services on their users.

During the course of one day, individuals and small groups of those present at the Sevenoaks Club were approached and asked if they would be prepared to share their views about the club and why they chose to come. All club members who were asked to participate, having been informed about the study on an earlier occasion, agreed to do so. The majority of respondents were interviewed in small groups of three or four, which were self-selected, whilst a four additional individual interviews took place. This reflected the natural groupings at the club on this occasion. The club co-ordinator and three volunteers were also interviewed. At each contact club a group interview involving all members attending for that session was carried out; this formed the major activity during the particular afternoon.

These individual and group interviews, which were all carried out during one specified week in November 1989, were characterized by a conversational approach, where respondents were encouraged to recount their experiences relatively freely and unprompted by the interviewer. In addition, the group discussions allowed individuals to share with each other their particular experiences, which prompted a considerable exchange of feelings and views about the service. As with the direct user and relative interviews reported in detail in Chapter 5, each interview was audio taped and extensive notes, but not full transcripts, were subsequently prepared, using as a framework the topics from the interview schedule.

In total, four group interviews and four individual interviews were conducted at the Sevenoaks Club. These involved a total of twenty respondents. At one contact club the group interviewed comprised ten users and three volunteers, and at the other sixteen users and four volunteers participated. Thus the findings presented here draw upon the views of fifty-three respondents.

Types of activity A similar overall structure or format to the afternoon was recognized by the users of both contact clubs. There was general agreement that the afternoon started with 'a cup of tea, a raffle and a chat', before some more organized activity took place: frequently a team quiz. Those who attended both clubs commented on the difference in space between the two locations, and how having a larger room provided more possibilities for breaking into smaller groups for part of the time. However, users of only one or other of the two clubs commented favourably on the social nature of each, and the opportunity for 'having a chat', 'airing your grievances', 'catching up with the news', and so on. The regular monthly outings from the Grove Club, organized by one volunteer, were also mentioned, along with enjoyable memories of annual summer and Christmas outings.

Like the users of the contact clubs, members of the Sevenoaks Club commented upon the opportunities for meeting people, having a chat, and generally being able to enjoy the company of others. They were, however, aware of a number of differences in the range of facilities available and the way in which the Sevenoaks Club was organized in a less formal way. Several comments were made about feeling part of a smaller sub-group within a larger friendly setting. This was seen as an advantage, as there were more opportunities for meeting people, whilst at the same time getting to know some people rather better. The meal also provided a focal point of the day for many members, who then stayed on, as one member explained:

> *... to have a chat and, if you want to after lunch ... get the cards out ... but [you're] never forced to do anything.*

This sense of being able to choose how to spend the time at the club was evident in a number of other comments; for example:

> *Sometimes we play cards, sometimes snooker ... [A member] sometimes organizes a small tournament.*

Sevenoaks Club members had heard about the opening of this drop-in centre in various ways, although most had heard either from a member of the Cosham team or from the nurse at the 'depot' clinic. A few had seen local posters inviting people to drop in, or had been encouraged to come along by a friend. Welcoming new members was a particular task undertaken by the volunteers, although often a member of the Cosham team might be involved in the initial introduction. For example, one member had appreciated being accompanied by his key-worker, a CPN, on his first visit:

> *I felt a bit reluctant, not knowing anyone. I'm glad I did go anyway ... have a good time and a laugh ... We play cards. It's really what you make it.*

Making contacts In commenting on opportunities for meeting people, users of all three clubs made the distinction between contacts with other users, with volunteers, and with staff. Some club attenders had made friends whom they met at other times during the week: sometimes by chance in the locality and on other occasions by arrangement. Another member referred to her friendship with a volunteer:

> *We struck up a friendship. We palled up through the club and found that we lived near each other. Now we meet outside of the club.*

In many ways, as the preceding quotation illustrates, users saw volunteers as friends, although they were well aware of the time that volunteers gave in getting to the club early and in preparing the lunchtime meal.

The volunteers also saw themselves as having a dual role, as one of them explained:

> *Being able to sit down and listen to people, to be there if someone wants to talk to me ... I enjoy that; also the busy time in the kitchen.*

Several volunteers were also aware of 'bridging the gap' between the direct users and the staff, as one volunteer ventured to explain:

> *We don't know all their problems ... like the staff do. We try to make people feel at home ... love and affection I suppose ... friendship.*

The co-ordinator of the Sevenoaks Club was seen by club members and volunteers as 'in charge'. This was mirrored in the co-ordinator's own view of her role:

> *An overview, being aware of everything that's going on and pulling it together, so that it's actually got some sense of organization ... and being around for volunteers and users.*

The OT helper was also seen as making a particular contribution at the Sevenoaks Club. Her ability to encourage people to participate in activities, whether it was playing snooker or getting a discussion group going, was commented upon by both users and volunteers. As one club member explained:

> *She's a lot of help: always here. She's very good with the youngsters ... getting into the activities. Nothing is too much trouble ... transport, shopping and so on.*

Access to professional support The need to maintain regular contact with professional staff was seen as important by users, volunteers and the co-ordinator. Users welcomed the opportunity to talk with a professionally qualified member of staff if they had some personal difficulties. Most were able to distinguish between the need for someone to talk to in a general way if they had difficulties, and when they needed access to more professional help. Club members generally felt that they could ask for this type of contact; for example, as one club member commented:

> *If I've got a problem about myself I will just ask: 'Have you got a few minutes?', when a member of staff calls in.*

This feeling that some members of staff would be calling in during the day was also important to the volunteers, who felt able to reassure any club member wanting to make contact.

The users were also aware that those staff members who initially had been involved in the setting up of the Sevenoaks Club now had less involvement in the club's day-to-day activities. As one club member commented:

> *They used to spend a lot of time here, but now it allows them time to go off and perhaps visit other clients who are housebound. The volunteers have relieved them a bit.*

The volunteers and co-ordinator also saw that staff members were now 'standing back from their previous involvement', but welcomed the level of ongoing support currently being offered. They appreciated the continued involvement of the OT helper and the knowledge that some back-up was available if needed from the duty officer at Acorn Lodge. This back-up was seen as:

> *... the important link ... but at the same time a feeling of being quite separate.*

They also commented on the professional staff's contribution to the overall management of the club, and their associated activities in fund-raising and service development.

The provision of staff cover was arranged slightly differently at the two contact clubs (see Chapter 2), although the comments made by those attending both were very similar, emphasizing their appreciation of regular access to a staff member, whether professionally qualified or not:

> *It's nice to have a member of staff here. Sometimes we're like the blind leading the blind here, aren't we?*

> *It's very important in case you feel a bit down. You can have a chat to a member of staff.*

Many of those interviewed chose to attend both contact clubs, and often the Sevenoaks Club as well. There was considerable variation in the way these facilities were used, and attenders appreciated both the range of available opportunities to meet people and the element of choice they had in attending one or more of these clubs.

Impact on users There was widespread agreement amongst those attending the contact clubs that the latter provided a place to go and meet others, as the following quotations illustrate:

> *Something to look forward to ... a cup of tea and a chat. It's the highlight of the week.*

> *It's company; someone to talk to and it gets you out and mixing.*

Similar comments were made by the Sevenoaks Club members, although they were more likely to refer to a wider range of activities and greater availability. For example:

> *Where I used to be shut in ... I know I went to [contact club] but that was only once a week ... it's brought me out in the open and now I'm only in one day a week. Otherwise I was stuck inside the four walls making myself worse. Here I'm mixing with people, talking, playing games, having a laugh and a joke. Otherwise at home I'd be either watching TV, playing records or sitting with things turning over inside, getting all up-tight, getting worked up and then having to go to see the doctor.*

A few club attenders were accompanied by their spouses. Opportunities to meet other people were much appreciated by carers, as one husband explained:

> *Getting out to bring the wife to the club means I can talk to other men.*

His coming to the club provided him with some relief from the continuous burden of caring, which he experienced as 'an invisible chain'.

Some club attenders more specifically emphasized their sense of belonging or feeling part of a group of people. 'Knowing somebody cares' was a recurring comment. As one regular attender explained:

> *Sometimes you make yourself go, because you know people will miss you, and when you go home you are glad you went because you enjoyed coming.*

This notion of either being missed or missing other regulars was a constant theme, primarily coming from those people attending the two contact clubs. The absence of a regular attender was generally discussed within the group; for example:

> *We ask if someone doesn't turn up and if someone hasn't been seen for a while. We might 'phone or ask the staff ... Part of coming here is checking the regular faces.*

For some club members, one important part of talking with others was the sense of a shared experience and of mutual support; for example:

> *... a great help to me ... I feel a lot better and don't get so depressed. I*

think it's because it's the same type of problem and I think mixing with people with the same problems helps a lot.

This view was shared by some of the volunteers, who had themselves experienced similar difficulties in the past, perhaps suggesting some blurring or overlapping of roles between user and volunteer. As one volunteer explained:

It's given me a sense of purpose since I retired ... There was no point in getting dressed to start with; now I'm very busy ...

Many of those interviewed had at some time attended both of the contact clubs and the Sevenoaks Club; this was evident from their comments about the different facilities. Whilst some differences were acknowledged, particularly in relation to the degree of structure and range of activity, all three clubs were seen as offering opportunities for meeting people and establishing friendships. Access to professional staff was also highly valued. The informality of the Sevenoaks Club appeared to provide greater flexibility and choice for its members, whereas those attending the contact clubs valued the familiarity of both the activities and a stable membership.

Overall, the users' views of the similarities and differences between the clubs broadly reflected those held by the members of the CCCG. This suggests a shared understanding of the ways in which the clubs operated, largely to provide opportunities for meeting others. The users interviewed were generally very positive about these facilities. Nevertheless, in expressing their satisfaction they were neither undiscerning in their comments nor unaware of changes over time. For example, the issue of access to professional support was an important one for many users. Whilst they valued their contacts with other users and volunteers, knowing that professional help was available if needed was also appreciated.

Summary

In the first part of this chapter we looked at some of the relationships between the Cosham Mental Health Service and the local social services area centre. Our study of the mental health work undertaken by staff based at the latter indicated areas of overlap between the two agencies, and raised questions about the ways in which mental health problems were being identified and referred to the most appropriate source of help. The second part of the chapter has explored another area of collaborative activity, that concerning the development of services for people with longer-term mental health problems, concluding with some users' views on these service initiatives.

The descriptive accounts of the setting up of a joint day care initiative, which involved several agencies, statutory and voluntary, and of the establishment Cosham Continuing Care Group, revealed how these developments had an impact on the professional practice of several team members. The shift from direct work with clients to service planning and management at a local level was highlighted, and this was subsequently confirmed by the perspectives of service users themselves. Several issues about the nature of the service, its priorities and possible future developments, and about working with others - professionals, volunteers and users - have been raised. Further exploration of these areas, with the emphasis primarily on professional practice, forms a substantial part of Chapter 6. First, however, we shall explore the more formal referral process and the characteristics of people with 'acute' problems seeking help from the service.

4 The boundaries of the service

Introduction

This chapter focuses on the more formal aspects of the referral process and how it evolved over the period of our study. It has two related aims; the first is to present basic information about a group of people newly referred to the Cosham Mental Health Service from the community during the period covered by our research. The second aim, which is inextricable from the first, is to examine the process by which these referrals for help were dealt with by the service. Issues then arise concerning the nature and boundaries of the service and its relationships with other local agencies.

With their emphasis on developing locally-based services, which were to be more accessible and more acceptable to their several users, an open referral system was regarded from the beginning as an essential feature of all the local teams in Portsmouth. Our account of the early development of the Cosham service indicated how the initial coming together of 'the community team' and 'the Vinten House team' represented a particular example of the need to co-ordinate the activities of various parts of an overall service. By the end of 1986, when the service had been in existence for several months, the co-ordination of overlapping areas of work undertaken with clients in the community by Vinten House staff and by staff based at North Lodge became a pressing concern, both for the service itself and for its main referrers, local GPs.

There was general agreement to the introduction of a regular 'referral meeting', at which referrals could be discussed and allocated within the whole team. In this way, all potential work to be undertaken in the community would be channelled to the service as a whole through a common referral system, regardless of to whom the work was initially directed or to whom it was subsequently allocated among the individual team members.

Broadly speaking, this system, once established, remained in operation throughout the two-year study reported here; in this chapter we seek to understand its operation. The referral meeting was normally attended by the majority of 'the community team', based at North Lodge during the pre-move period of the research and subsequently at Acorn Lodge, and by at least one representative of the staff of the residential unit, usually the Clinical Manager, during each of the pre-, partial and post-move periods. As was evident from our descriptive account of the service, the referral meeting became a prominent and regular feature of Monday mornings at North Lodge and subsequently of Wednesday mornings at Acorn Lodge.

The referral process

A preliminary view of the referral process

To begin to understand the operation of the referral meeting, a preliminary analysis was carried out of new referrals made to the team via these meetings during the nine-month period July 1987 - March 1988 inclusive, using as the sole source of information the so-called 'referral book'. In this book, basic details of each new referral had been recorded by administrative staff in date order, along with the date of the meeting at which the referral had been discussed and the initial allocation decision taken, i.e. the name of the person by whom further work was to be carried out.

The referral book also indicated whether a person referred was entirely new to the service, or had had previous contact. The operational definition which we have used in what follows relates to this system. We have defined a new referral as any referral where the person concerned was not currently being helped and had no recorded contact with the service (i.e. had not been current on a team member's caseload) during the preceding six months, whether or not they had had contact during an earlier period. Our primary points of reference are referral incidents, not the individuals involved; just as each entry in the referral book represents an incident rather than a person. An individual person can in principle appear more than once in the book (and in our analysis), but a referral is a 'one-off' event.

It is important to keep in mind that the data presented here specifically exclude direct inpatient admissions, both to Vinten House and to the Intensive Care Unit (Brunel Villa). Ongoing work with 'continuing care' clients is also excluded by definition. Some of the people included here may of course later have become, or may yet become, recipients of longer-term help, just as they may also have (or may have already had) a period of inpatient care.

The first four tables present basic data for the nine-month period to the end of March 1988. New referrals made from July 1987 to March 1988 are examined by month, source of referral, and initial allocation within the team; all as recorded in the referral book. Table 4.1 shows that there were 208 new referrals in the nine-month period, and that they appear to have settled into a reasonably steady month-by-month flow, with a lull around Christmas. Of these referrals, 83 per cent were made by GPs. 82 per cent of these GP referrals were made by letter.

Table 4.1
Monthly new referrals, July 1987/March 1988

July	Aug	Sept	Oct	Nov	Dec	Jan	Feb	Mar	Total
14	17	31	23	27	16	25	30	25	208

Table 4.2 shows the initial allocation of these new referrals amongst the various team members, as recorded in the referral book. This pattern of allocation over the whole nine-month period was mirrored, broadly speaking, month-by-month, with numbers in each group being roughly stable proportions of the monthly totals of referrals.

Table 4.2
Initial allocation

Psychiatrists (incl locums, registrars etc)	64
Community psychiatric nurses (CPNs)	72
Psychologist	14
Social worker	8
Occupational therapists	8
Vinten House staff	35
Other (eg Alcohol or Drug Services, SSD)	7
Total	208

An open referral system implies that GPs and others refer to the team rather than, as traditionally, the only route being from GP to consultant psychiatrist. Thus there is the possibility of direct access to various members of the team and therefore of direct access to a range of services, rather than an initial outpatient appointment with a psychiatrist being the routine response. Nevertheless, the preliminary analysis of new referrals from the community during the nine months around the time our research began, presented in Table 4.2, shows a substantial number of new referrals initially being seen by doctors.

Despite the institution of the referral meeting, 31 per cent of the new referrals in the nine months to the end of March 1988 were first dealt with by the consultant, a locum, or a junior doctor, compared with 35 per cent by CPNs and 17 per cent by Vinten House staff. This pattern holds if we focus on only the last six months of this period, up to the end of March, the equivalent percentages being 29, 32 and 19 and the numerical differences being largely a reflection of the psychologist only featuring from September.

Additional features of the referral process

The referral book for this period contained two further types of entry. One variant indicated that in addition to the presentation of new referrals, the referral meeting was also providing an opportunity for individual members of the team to bring cases back for further discussion, leading to possible additional involvement on the part of colleagues or reallocation within the team. Entries recording this showed which team member had brought the case back to the meeting.

The other entries not recording new referrals also indicated that the person concerned had been discussed at a referral meeting on a certain date, and suggested that the instigator was a professional from outside the team. It was not clear on the basis of the information in the book whether this group could be considered as having been re-referred to the service in a formal sense. However, like that group of cases brought back to a meeting by team members, the people concerned appeared to be already known, in that each had been recorded as newly-referred in the quite recent past.

Thus we can begin to understand that what has been called 'the referral meeting' involved more than preliminary discussion of new referrals from the community. Seeking a preliminary understanding of the pattern and processing of referrals to the service already leads us to see the referral book as essentially a brief record of all individual clients discussed at each referral meeting, rather than as simply a record of new referrals to the service from 'outside' in a straightforward sense.

We examined the entries which suggested these two additional dimensions of the referral meeting which we have now introduced to our account. Table 4.3 shows the sources of both types of referral back to the meeting, and their subsequent (re)allocation. Both overall and consistently month-by-month, team psychiatrists were responsible for over 50 per cent of the instances where cases came back to the meeting. Two-thirds of the psychiatrists' cases included here were also brought back during the first five of the nine months analyzed in the table. Particularly in the early months, GPs re-referred a number of people. Overall numbers in other groups are very small.

Table 4.3
Cases brought back to referral meetings for review

Brought back by team members:		
	psychiatrists	38
	CPNs	2
	OTs	0
	psychologist	0
	social worker	8
	Vinten House staff	1
Sub-total		49
Brought back by others:		
	GPs	12
	other hospital staff	4
	self	3
	family	1
	other	1
Sub-total		21
Total		70

Those cases brought back by team psychiatrists had received an initial medical assessment. The information in Table 4.4 suggests that after review by the team these cases were (re)allocated to other members, mainly CPNs and to a lesser extent Vinten House staff. As Table 4.4 also shows, the doctors did, however, continue with some of these cases and/or were allocated others as a result of review by the team as a whole.

Table 4.4
(Re)allocation upon review

(Re)allocated to team members:		
	psychiatrists	12
	CPNs	33
	OTs	1
	psychologist	1
	social worker	7
	Vinten House staff	11
Sub-total		65
(Re)allocated to other services		2
No further action		3
Total		70

This somewhat crude analysis, based solely on data from the referral book, does give some indication of how the referral meeting was operating in dealing with new referrals to the service from the community. Initial allocation was clearly only the beginning of a process which requires closer examination, first through more detailed study of a sample of new referrals, then by examining the subsequent use made of the service by some of these clients.

Patterns of referral over one year

The remainder of this chapter takes a closer look at new referrals over a continuous period of twelve months within our overall study period. The data presented were extracted and collated retrospectively at two quite separate points in time. One set of data covers the six-month period from April 1st until September 30th 1988: the six-month period immediately following that upon which the foregoing sketch has been based. The second covers the next subsequent six-month period: from October 1st 1988 until March 31st 1989.

These two six-month periods were deliberately chosen at the outset of our research to enable a comparison between the patterns of referral over a substantial period of time (one year), with the date at which the projected move of the service to its base in Cosham itself falling almost exactly at the mid-point. Without therefore prejudging what the impact of that move would be, we would be able to observe and assess any such impact on the types of client referred and the process by which new referrals were dealt with.

As readers by now know, the move did not in fact take place as we and others had envisaged. Only part of the service moved its base to Acorn Lodge in October 1988, with the staff of the residential facility, Vinten House, remaining on the main hospital site until the following June. We were thus confronted with three broad time periods instead of two, with an interim partial move phase between the pre-move and post-move phases around which we had made our research plans. Whilst we present a variety of data on all three of these phases in this book, because of the important linkage between the data we sought on new referrals and the cohort of clients from whom we wished to draw our interview sample, we decided to adhere to our original time plan and not to collect and analyze data on new referrals for that (reduced) proportion of our agreed study period when the whole Cosham service was based at Acorn Lodge. Therefore, in relation to the discussion in Chapter 2, where the activity data presented referred to pre-move and post-move periods, readers should keep in mind that the two periods for which referral data are presented in the present chapter reflect pre-move and partial move situations respectively.

In the present chapter, and with this particular data, we are only concerned to analyze the process of using the service as far as the first direct contact or, where none appears to have been made, attempted contact, with the client by a team member, following the referral concerned. In order to examine the subsequent use made of the various parts of the service by a cohort of clients over an appropriate period of time it is obviously necessary for sufficient time to have elapsed following referral to permit a comprehensive and systematic view. We have conducted such an analysis, using clients drawn as part of our interview sample from the second six-month period for which referral data are presented here. This material appears in Chapter 5.

We have drawn upon case-files in addition to the referral book to study the process by which contact was sought with the client in order further to assess and negotiate the most appropriate form of help which might be provided. If there was an apparent contradiction between a case-file and the referral book we have given preference to the file, assuming the book simply to have recorded a preliminary decision which quite possibly was overtaken by subsequent events.

We have examined data for each of the two six-month periods, April 1st to September 30th 1988, and October 1st 1988 to March 31st 1989. Where appropriate the tables and discussion which follow present and discuss the data for each period separately, highlighting any significant differences and indicating changes over time or at particular points. However, where analysis has revealed no such significant features we simply present composite data covering the whole twelve months from April 1988 to March 1989.

We have reported that the data were extracted and analyzed at two distinct points in time. This may have introduced larger than normal coding variations. We should also mention here that data for the first six months were analyzed manually and for the second six months using the computer package SNAP; the latter approach was quicker but in some respects less flexible than the former. Consequently we have had to 'smooth' some differences in coding at certain points when combining the two data sets. We do not believe that any major patterns are likely to have been either obscured or artificially created by this.

Once again it is important to remember that the picture given here of how the service dealt with new referrals from the community does not represent the team's total workload at any point in time. Specifically excluded are direct inpatient admissions, including those to Vinten House, and ongoing work with existing clients in the community, including any continuing contact commencing prior to the period analyzed.

Age and sex of twelve months' new referrals

For the period from 1st April to 30th September 1988, the referral book records 166 new referrals to the Cosham team; for the period 1st October 1988 to 31st March 1989 it records 169 new referrals: a remarkably similar figure. To remind readers, our primary points of reference are referral incidents, not the individuals involved, and a 'new referral' is defined as a referral where the person concerned had had no contact with the service during the preceding six months, whether or not they had had contact prior to that.

Three individuals appeared in the referral book as new referrals on two separate occasions during the first six-month period analyzed: i.e. not once as a new referral and later as brought back to the team for review/further discussion in the manner already outlined. This could be simply a matter of recording errors or inconsistencies on the part of the service. There were no similar examples in the second six-month period. For the most part in what follows we simply present data on the basis of 335 referral incidents which involved 332 different individuals in the overall twelve-month period. Where necessary, we refer to 166 referral incidents, involving 163 different individuals, and/or 169 referral incidents, involving 169 different individuals, in what hereafter we shall often refer to as the 'first period' and the 'second period' respectively.

Of the 166 incidents recorded as new referrals during the first period, fifty-four (33%) concerned men and 112 (67%) women. Table 4.5.1 shows the age and sex breakdown of the individuals referred, age being calculated in full years at the date of the referral incident. The group contains twice as many women as men. Just over one-third of the first period's new referrals were of people aged less than thirty years, just over one-fifth over fifty, and the rest - nearly half - were aged between thirty and fifty. Over 40 per cent of the 166 referrals were of women aged between thirty and sixty years of age.

Table 4.5.1
Age and sex of new referrals (4/88 - 9/88)

Age	Male	Female	Total
under 20	7	6	13
20-29	17	29	46
30-39	12	31	43
40-49	5	23	28
50-59	7	16	23
60 & over	6	7	13
Total	54	112	166

During the second period, there were 169 referral incidents. Fifty-nine (35%) involved men and 110 (65%) involved women. Table 4.5.2 shows the age and sex breakdown of this group, which as in the previous six months contains roughly twice as many women as men. The people referred in the second period were slightly younger overall than those referred in the first period, with 40 per cent aged under thirty and only 15 per cent aged fifty or more.

Table 4.5.2
Age and sex of new referrals (10/88 - 3/89)

Age	Male	Female	Total
under 20	3	9	12
20-29	20	36	56
30-39	16	33	49
40-49	8	18	26
50-59	11	7	18
60 & over	1	7	8
Total	59	110	169

Looking at these trends in a little more detail, the main changes were an increase in the twenty to twenty-nine age band, especially of women, whose numbers and percentages were also up a little in the under twenty and thirty to thirty-nine bands. There were decreases in the numbers and proportions of women in the fifty to fifty-nine and sixty and over age groups. The numbers and proportions of men were up slightly in the second period in all age bands except the under twenties and the over sixties. Once again, almost half of the second group of referrals were of people aged between thirty and fifty, with 34 per cent of the 169 being of women aged between thirty and sixty.

Marital status

Roughly 60 per cent of the people referred during the twelve months for which referral data were analyzed were recorded as either being married or cohabiting, whilst almost 40 per cent were single, widowed or divorced/separated. Tables 4.6 and 4.7 show the information on marital status over the whole twelve months, broken down by age and sex respectively.

Nothing particularly noteworthy appears from the variation of marital status with age within the overall group of twelve months' new referrals. However, the sex distribution in relation to marital status does have some interesting features. There are numerically equal numbers of single women and single men in the group, despite the 2:1 overall female:male ratio. Less marked, but also worthy of comment, is the 3:1 ratio of women:men in the married sub-group. This reflects a well-documented national picture; overall rates of mental illness are higher for women than for men, and this bias is more pronounced amongst married than single women (Miles, 1987).

Table 4.6
Age by marital status of new referrals (4/88 - 3/89)

Age	Sgle	Marr	Cohab	Wid	Div/sep	Not recd	Total
under 20	23	1	1	0	0	0	25
20-29	44	41	8	0	5	4	102
30-39	14	66	3	0	6	3	92
40-49	3	41	2	0	6	2	54
50-59	5	27	0	2	3	4	41
60 & over	1	13	0	2	1	4	21
Total	90	189	14	4	21	17	335

There was a slight increase in the number (10) of single people referred in the second period, and a corresponding rise of 5.5 per cent in their proportional representation in the overall group. Most of this increase (7) was made up of women.

Numerically speaking, women are over-represented in the widowed and divorced/separated sub-groups relative to the 2:1 sex division of the overall group, perhaps reflecting that the women in the overall sample, especially those referred during the first six-month period, tend to be older as a group than the men.

Table 4.7
Sex by marital status of new referrals (4/88 - 3/89)

Sex	Sgle	Marr	Cohab	Wid	Div/sep	Not recd	Total
male	45	48	4	0	5	11	113
female	45	141	10	4	16	6	222
Total	90	189	14	4	21	17	335

The proportion of people who have experienced divorce may not be fairly represented here, since recorded relationships may have been new/current stable ones following earlier marital breakdown. With current patterns and attitudes in a state of flux, recorded formal marital status may not reflect accurately either with whom a person lives or from whom they draw emotional support. If original data were being collected, as opposed to extracting from brief case records, it would be preferable to seek a fuller picture of actual relationships rather than formal civil status.

Month of referral

Table 4.8 shows the month-by-month pattern of new referrals from April 1988 to March 1989. This was relatively stable, fluctuating around an average of about twenty-eight per month. Thus the level of new referrals continued over a further twelve months at a broadly similar level to that established in the initial period (shown in Table 4.1), once the local service had become established.

Table 4.8
Monthly new referrals, April 1988/March 1989

Apr	May	Jun	Jul	Aug	Sep	Oct	Nov	Dec	Jan	Feb	Mar	Total
36	21	26	32	27	24	19	32	22	31	36	29	335

We have used the date when team discussion took place at an allocation meeting (or of immediate action in response to an urgent referral), rather than strictly the date of referral, as our reference point. With allocation meetings taking place on Mondays during the first period, some of the fluctuation which is evident may have been a result of the incidence of Public Holidays. October's partial move to Acorn Lodge and the Christmas break in December are also reflected. If December is excluded, there appears to be a higher level of new referrals sustained over four of the last five months of the period analyzed. Whilst this could be a significant trend, looking back to Table 4.1 suggests that there may be an annual pattern, with a higher level of new referrals in the winter months.

Previous contact with the Cosham service

We have defined new referrals as involving people who had not been in direct contact with the service during a six-month period prior to the referral incident concerned. Of our sample group of 166 new referrals made during the April/September period of 1988, fifty-six (34%) were of people previously known to the service, i.e. who had had contact during a period more than six months prior to their present referral. 107 (64%) were of people not previously known in this sense. The remaining three referrals were the second incidents involving the three people referred twice during the period.

Of the 169 new referrals during the period October 1988/March 1989, the corresponding figures were fifty-four (32%) previously known and 114 (67%) not previously in contact. An overall pattern of roughly one in three referrals being of someone who had had previous contact with the service, but had not been in contact during the preceding six months, was thus sustained over the full twelve months analyzed. However, whilst this pattern was approximately mirrored on a month-by-month basis during most of this period, there was some increase over the last few months of the second six-month period in the proportion of new referrals which were of people previously known to the service.

Table 4.9
Age and sex of people previously known to the service (4/88 - 3/89)

Age	Male	Female	Total
under 20	4	3	7
20-29	10	9	19
30-39	12	24	36
40-49	3	16	19
50-59	4	13	17
60 & over	4	8	12
Total	37	73	110

Table 4.9 examines the age and sex breakdown of the 110 people who were newly referred - in the sense we have defined this - between April 1988 and March 1989, but who had had contact during a previous period. There appears little to distinguish those people known to the service before the referral concerned from the overall referral group, and therefore from those people referred for the first time during the period. Although Table 4.9 does not reveal this, the slightly changed age and sex profile of the overall group of new referrals for the second six-month period (see Tables 4.5.1 and 4.5.2) is reflected when figures on earlier contact are considered for the two six-month periods separately. Overall however, there is a somewhat predictable tendency for those people in the older age groups to be a little more likely to have had previous contact with the service.

Source of referral

Over the whole twelve months for which data were analyzed, 88 per cent of new referrals (294 out of 335), were made by local general practitioners. There was only a very slight fall in this proportion in the second six months as compared with the first: from 90 per cent to 85 per cent. Table 4.10 shows this, along with the sources of the other new referrals to the service during the period studied. There was some broadening in the range of referral sources over the second six months, including an increase in the number - still very small however - of self-referrals. Health visitors were the most prominent new group of professional referrers. There was also an increase in referrals from consultant physicians, and there were referrals from a wider range of social work contexts, although the level of referral from the local social services area centre remained very low. The slight broadening of referral sources, coupled with the decrease in referrals from other teams, suggests a gradually increasing understanding of the service across the city.

Although each referral has been coded to a single source, there was evidence of more than one professional having been involved in a referral

Table 4.10
Source of referral

	4/88-9/88	10/88-3/89	4/88-3/89
GPs	150	144	294
Health visitors	0	6	6
Other Portsmouth Mental Health Teams	5	1	6
Queen Alexandra Hospital	3	2	5
Consultant physicians	1	4	5
Northern Road Drug Advice Centre	2	0	2
Havant Day Hospital	0	1	1
Consultant psychiatrist outside District	1	0	1
Social Services Dept area centre	3	1	4
Naval Welfare Service	0	2	2
Social workers - child & family therapy	0	1	1
Probation officers	0	1	1
Self-referrals	1	6	7
Total	166	169	335

in some cases. For example, a small number of the referrals by GPs had also involved a local social worker contacting a client's doctor, whilst some of the self-referrals were at a GP's suggestion. This is more fully explored in subsequent chapters via interview data.

Method of referral

Table 4.11 shows that over 70 per cent of the new referrals during the twelve months analyzed came to the team by letter, usually on the official form for a GP referral to a hospital service.

Table 4.11
Method of referral

	4/88-9/88	10/88-3/89	4/88-3/89
Letter	122	117	239
Telephone	37	40	77
Memo	5	4	9
'Bleep'	1	0	1
'Drop-in'	0	3	3
Not recorded	1	5	6
Total	166	169	335

Most of the other referrals were made by telephone, except some of those in a sense internal to the local hospital services, including for example those from the other Portsmouth Community Mental Health

Teams and the District Drug Service, whose own referral forms were often used and are included collectively as 'memos'. Telephone referrals were often followed with written information.

Examining the pattern of referral methods month-by-month over the first of our two six-month periods revealed something of a shift over time from GP letters to telephone contacts, perhaps giving an early indication of increasing familiarity and decreasing formality among the various professionals involved. However, whilst comparing the second six months as a whole with the first also suggests such a trend, it is so slight that instances where the method of referral was not recorded could negate it. Month-by-month examination over the second six months revealed no evident trend away from the predominance of formal GP referrals by letter.

With self- or family referrals featuring very rarely during the first six months, it was hardly surprising to find no 'drop-in' referrals, which as we have reported elsewhere (Powell and Lovelock, 1987a) became increasingly common during the development of the District's community-based services for drug misusers, situated nearby. The small increase in self-referrals in the second period is reflected in a small(er) increase in the number of 'drop-ins'.

Reason for referral

It is notoriously difficult to categorize 'reasons for referral' adequately (Phillips et al., 1988), not least because the referrer and the person being referred - to name but two of the parties concerned - may have different perceptions of the process (Smith and Cantley, 1985). To attempt to understand the reasons which referrers had for referring the people concerned to the team, we have drawn on information held in case files. Mainly this comprised letters from GPs - sometimes quite long and frequently discursive - together with notes of telephone conversations. What we offer here is an interpretation of this written information.

For our purposes the most significant elements contained in the various referral communications can be grouped as follows:

(i) references to basic sources or causes of the mental distress being experienced by the client;

(ii) specific symptoms for which specialist help was seen as appropriate and necessary;

(iii) views about suitable forms of treatment or help which the team could possibly provide.

For ease of presentation we shall deal with each of these three elements separately, although they necessarily overlap and were often intertwined in our source material. Within each of these broad groupings a number of more specific items were mentioned by referrers with varying regularity. Whilst we have created and labelled the overall groupings, we would emphasize that the more specific items directly relate to the terms employed in the written referral information.

(i) Stated sources and causes of distress Table 4.12 shows the frequency with which a number of types or areas of difficulty were mentioned by referrers as sources of the problems being experienced by the people they were referring for specialist help.

Table 4.12
Reason for referral - sources/causes of distress

	4/88-9/88	10/88-3/89	4/88-3/89
Relationship problems	38	52	90
Life events	23	39	62
Illness/disability/accident	8	4	12
Practical difficulties (eg £, accommodn)	7	3	10
Other	0	2	2
Total (mentions)	76	100	176
Nothing of this kind recorded (cases)	98	84	182
(Number of new referrals in period	166	169	335)

The most common grouping was 'relationship problems', with ninety mentions over the twelve-month period studied. This includes (in decreasing frequency) references to difficulties with spouses or cohabitees, children or 'the family', and in work relationships, along with such things as 'lacking confidence', 'feels isolated', and 'communication problems'. 'Life events' were the second most commonly referred-to group of factors (sixty-two mentions). Among specific experiences mentioned under this heading as sources of mental ill health, again in decreasing order of frequency, were divorce or the breakdown of long-standing relationships, bereavements involving various people close to the client, and varied problems seen as stemming from traumas in giving birth and in one case from termination of a pregnancy. There were also single instances of a reference to being a victim of child abuse, of recent release from prison, and of a court case pending. A recent change of address was mentioned in three cases, not as in itself problematic but as a ground for referral in the light of previous and/or ongoing mental health difficulties. Two less common groups of factors were also evident: worries about a serious illness or problems about coping with the consequences of accidents or disabilities, and various difficulties with financial or housing matters.

Tables 4.12, 4.13 and 4.14 each simply indicate how often one or another factor was mentioned in the recorded referral information. In so far as the items relate to individual people referred they often do so as one of a group of factors acknowledged, including in some cases two variants of the same sort of difficulty. Strictly therefore, Table 4.12 reports that in the period April to September 1988 seventy-six sources of distress of the broad kinds indicated were recorded in referral letters etc., shared among sixty-eight referral incidents. In the period October 1988 to March 1989, one hundred such sources of distress were similarly shared among eighty-five referral incidents.

Given that referral information in respect of the two six-month periods was extracted and analyzed separately, we should acknowledge that the apparent increase in the number of items mentioned in relation to the second six months' new referrals could reflect that more information was being given by GPs and other referrers and/or that more was extracted and coded by the researchers. In addition, as mentioned earlier, the analysis of data for the first six-month period was carried out manually, whereas that for the second period was done using the computer package SNAP. Whilst the former was more flexible, the latter was quicker and greatly assisted more detailed examination of patterns. As far as possible we used the categories devised in analyzing the first period's new referrals when analyzing the later data. However, it is in this section that variations in the application of coding categories as between data for the two six-month periods is most likely. Only the broad trends evident should therefore be regarded as significant. In addition, we had to adopt a different means of dealing with the phenomenon of multiple reasons for referral being recorded in particular cases under any of our groupings of reasons.

An impression was gained whilst extracting and coding this data, of an increased frequency (still not high) of references to clients' views during the second period, and likewise of some gender differentiation among recorded reasons for referral of the sort being considered here. Although we were only able to examine this for the second six months, women, and especially women in the 30-49 age band, tend to be 'over-represented' amongst the group recorded as having 'relationship problems' as a source of distress. Most of the men for whom this was mentioned were aged 20-39. In respect of 'life events', men were 'over-represented' in the 30-60 age band and women in the 20-29 group.

(ii) Psychiatric symptoms as reasons for seeking specialist help Table 4.13 shows the main terms used by referrers in this context. 'Anxiety', 'depression' (whether seen as clinical or not), and frequently both in combination as 'anxious and depressed', were overwhelmingly the most commonly recorded 'symptoms' in GP letters and other referral documentation

throughout the twelve-month period, being mentioned 100 times in relation to the first six months' new referrals and 131 times in the context of the second.

Table 4.13
Reason for referral - psychiatric symptoms

	4/88-9/88	10/88-3/89	4/88-3/89
Anxiety and/or depression	100	131	231
Agoraphobia (anx/depr not also mentioned)	6	8	14
Other phobias (.. .. ..)	3	1	4
Psychosomatic problems (.. .. ..)	3	9	12
Hypochondria (.. .. ..)	1	2	3
Eating disorders	8	3	11
Psychosexual problems	5	3	8
Substance abuse	7	3	10
Overdose or suicidal (tendencies)	10	10	20
Aggressive/temper tantrums	6	5	11
Schizophrenic illness	2	4	6
Paranoia	1	0	1
Request for formal psychiatric assessment/ review (incl urgent home visit)	31	7	38
Request for psychological assessment	7	5	12
Request for nurse/CPN assesst/involvement	2	1	3
Request for assessment by team (member)	4	3	7
Other	6	3	9
Total (mentions)	202	198	400
Nothing of this kind recorded (cases)	20	28	48
(Number of new referrals in period	166	169	335)

In a number of cases a specific request for a specialist assessment (notably a formal psychiatric assessment) had apparently been a major reason for referral. Sometimes this was the only such reason recorded; sometimes it appeared along with a reference to specific symptoms or with one or more of the other sorts of statement considered in sub-sections *(i)* or *(iii)*. There appears to have been a reduction in the frequency of requests for formal psychiatric assessment during the second period analyzed, which has not been 'balanced' by requests for assessment by other specified team members or by the team as a whole.

In analyzing the case file material we have subsumed such terms as 'distressed' and 'disturbed', 'panic attacks' and 'sleeping difficulties', within this category where, as was often the case, this seemed to be the sense of recorded statements. In Table 4.13 we have also used 'anxious and/or depressed' as an over-riding category for a number of conditions such as agoraphobia where the latter were mentioned in addition to a general reference to anxiety or depression. Where these same conditions were referred to without explicit additional mention of anxiety and/or depression they have been recorded more specifically in the table. Thus psychosomatic disorders of various sorts, and to a lesser extent agoraphobia, were rather more common features of clients' distress than would appear from a first glance at the table, since both were frequently mentioned as part of an account of a general anxiety state. Certain other conditions, such as eating disorders and psychosexual problems, have been specifically recorded in the table for all cases where they were mentioned, whether or not anxiety and/or depression were also noted. If this latter was the case, both the specific disorder and 'anxiety and/or depression' have been 'scored'.

During the first six-month period, April/September 1988, there were 202 recorded mentions of reasons for referral categorized by the researchers as 'symptoms', shared between 146 referral incidents. In the second period, October 1988/March 1989, there were 198 such mentions, amongst 141 referral incidents. There was nothing recorded relevant to this category as a whole in only twenty instances during the first period and in twenty-eight in the second.

As in the previous sub-section, potential methodological differences make caution necessary in considering any differences between and within categories as between the two six-month periods; the overall balance, especially the predominance of 'anxiety and/or depression', is the most significant finding.

(iii) Referrers' 'prescriptions'/recommendations In about a quarter of cases, referrers offered a suggestion for the form of help they felt might be appropriate for the Cosham service to give to the client concerned. Details are shown in Table 4.14. Forty-one such 'prescriptions' were offered in respect of thirty-nine referrals in the first six-month period, and forty-eight relating to forty-two referrals in the second. Only in eight cases overall were two possible forms of help suggested.

Given their sources, predominantly GPs' letters of referral, the data presented in this section as a whole not only provide a picture of the range of difficulties being experienced by the people referred for help, but also indicate referrers' perceptions of mental health problems and how they might be ameliorated, in particular by the Cosham Mental Health Team. Some referrers might be more prone than others to refer to a specialist service, and/or to offer suggestions for potential ways of helping. In examining referral letters, we noticed that particular GPs had particular styles, used particular forms of words, and perhaps tended to focus on particular types of problem.

Even more than in the two foregoing subsections, several of the categories used here clearly overlap. The terms employed are those of the referrers, any two of whom may perhaps use different 'labels' to indicate similar thoughts. The specific patterning of suggestions between categories and over time suggested by Table 4.14 is probably not of great significance, but it undoubtedly reflects referrers' perceptions and expectations of the service.

Table 4.14
Reason for referral - referrers' 'prescriptions'

	4/88-9/88	10/88-3/89	4/88-3/89
Counselling/behaviour modification	10	20	30
Anxiety management group	10	4	14
Support/ongoing monitoring	6	4	10
Psychological help/treatment	5	2	7
CPN involvement	4	4	8
Psychotherapy	2	1	3
Relaxation	2	5	7
Women's group	1	0	1
'Depot' clinic	1	0	1
Social support/someone to talk to	0	6	6
Carer/family needs help	0	2	2
Total (mentions)	41	48	89
No recommendation recorded (cases)	127	127	254
(Number of new referrals in period	166	169	335)

Impressionistically at least, there was a slightly increased likelihood (still not very great) of finding references to clients' - and/or in a handful of cases, carers' - expressed wishes or views in the referral information for the second six-month period analyzed.

The category 'counselling/behaviour modification' contains, especially in the second period, a number of references to more specific forms of help, such as marital, psychosexual, and grief counselling.

It appears that perceptions and expectations of the service not only varied between individuals, but were subject to change over time, in the context of the two-way process of feedback and direct interaction between the Cosham team and local GPs and other referrers. It seems reasonable to assume that thereby clarification took place about what constitutes an appropriate referral to the service. This issue was explored in our interviews with GPs, reported in Chapter 5.

Psychiatric diagnosis

A formal psychiatric diagnosis was sometimes included within the referral information held in case files. Sometimes this was offered by a referring GP, perhaps implicitly or explicitly seeking confirmation of her/his own assessment. Alternatively, an earlier diagnosis may have been mentioned, perhaps made by a psychiatrist in another area or some time ago. Any such statements have already been used in sub-section *(ii)* concerning 'symptoms' as reasons for referral. Table 4.15 gives a specific analysis of all formal diagnoses recorded in the case files of people newly referred during the twelve-month period analyzed, including both those earlier diagnoses just mentioned and any made subsequent to the referral process, which it was therefore not appropriate to include earlier. These latter diagnoses were mostly made by psychiatrists on domiciliary visits or at outpatient assessments or reviews, either in direct response to the referral concerned or within the subsequent few months.

Table 4.15
Psychiatric diagnosis

Depressive illness	9
Depression + anorexia	1
Anxiety + depression	6
Anxiety state	5
Anxiety + phobia	3
Agoraphobia	8
Hypochondria	3
Anorexia	1
Schizophrenic illness	4
Personality disorder	4
Psychological reaction	2
Not clinically depressed	2
Not psychiatrically ill	1
Total (mentions)	49
No diagnosis recorded (cases)	287
(Number of new referrals in period	335)

In twenty-seven individual cases during the first and twenty-one cases in the second six-month period analyzed, a formal psychiatric diagnosis was recorded on the case-files held by the team as having been made at some time. The table includes three 'negative diagnoses', all during the first period; in two of these cases it was stated in the context of an assessment after referral that the person concerned was not clinically depressed, whilst in the other case a referring consultant from another area stated that the client was not psychiatrically ill. One of the people stated not to be clinically depressed on formal assessment had been diagnosed (presumably appropriately) as suffering from a depressive illness at an earlier stage. This 'double count' explains why the table sums to forty-nine.

A little under half of the forty-eight individual clients involved were already known to the Cosham service at the time of the referral concerned: twelve of twenty-seven (44%) during the first six-month period and ten of twenty-one (48%) during the second.

Response to referrals

In considering the referral process, our background assumption thus far has been that, following a referral, discussion first took place among the team at the weekly 'referral meeting', where a preliminary view was arrived at, representing the team members' shared perspective on the most appropriate course of action. A member of the team was then given responsibility for contacting the client, in order to make a more detailed assessment and negotiate what form(s) of help might be most appropriate and acceptable.

Whilst this remained the predominant pattern of response on the part of the Cosham service throughout the period covered by our research, more detailed study of all new referrals made during the twelve-month period April 1988/March 1989, including an analysis of the case files of the people concerned, revealed that in some instances an immediate response was made as a matter of urgency and in advance of a team discussion at the referral meeting. As we shall see later, a proportion of the referrals which received urgent attention were then discussed subsequently, often very soon, in a referral meeting.

Urgent action in response to referrals As Table 4.16 shows, very similar proportions of new referrals received a response in advance of full team discussion in each of the two six-month periods for which separate analyses were carried out. The nature of these responses and the actors making them on behalf of the service were also relatively constant over the full twelve months studied in detail.

There were thirty-seven instances (11%) in the period April 1988/March 1989 where some form of action was taken prior to a team discussion. The remaining 298 (89%) new referrals received initial attention by means of discussion by the team, usually within a week of referral.

Overall, during the twelve-month period analyzed, there was no significant patterning in respect of the age or sex of those people newly referred (as we have defined this) and receiving an urgent response.

Similarly, the proportions of new referrals which received an urgent response and which involved people previously known to the Cosham service, and the sources of these referrals, reflected the relevant patterns within the overall sample.

Table 4.16
Initial response in advance of team meeting

	4/88-9/88	10/88-3/89	4/88-3/89
Domiciliary visit by consultant	5	5	10
Home visit by non-medical team member	6	4	10
Seen as outpatient (by a psychiatrist)	3	1	4
Assessment following overdose	2	1	3
Assessment at general hospital	1	0	1
Admission to Vinten House	1	0	1
Seen by duty therapist at Vinten House	0	2	2
Offered appointment at Vinten House	0	1	1
Seen by duty officer at Acorn Lodge	n/a	3	3
Seen at health centre	0	0	0
Referred to family therapy team	0	1	1
Out of area - transfer	1	0	1
Sub-total	19	18	37
Initial discussion at team meeting	147	151	298
Total	166	169	335

Table 4.16 also indicates the course of action taken in those cases where an immediate response to a referral was deemed necessary. A significant point about the sub-group of thirty-seven referrals where action was taken in advance of team discussion, is that they included six actual or feared suicide attempts and sixteen formal requests for psychiatric assessment. If the resultant domiciliary visits made by the consultant or a locum (not made in all such cases), and assessments carried out at local general hospitals, are taken together with outpatient appointments, we can see that urgent action by medical members of the team accounted for almost half of the immediate responses made during the period April 1988/March 1989.

Table 4.17 indicates specifically which team members were involved in immediate responses. The relative prominence of Vinten House staff in both six-month periods in respect of urgent action is worthy of note. This may well reflect the twenty-four-hour availability of cover at Vinten and the fact that from August 1988 there was an integrated duty system involving the whole Cosham team, with liaison between the duty therapist at Vinten and the other member of the overall team on duty.

Taking Tables 4.16 and 4.17 together, there is little numerically significant change in the nature and balance of responses prior to a full team discussion as between the two six-month periods. There is a slight decrease in home visits by team members other than psychiatrists, in favour of duty staff seeing people either at Acorn Lodge or Vinten House, including in two cases in response to a client 'dropping in'.

Table 4.17
Actors responding to referral in advance of team meeting

	4/88-9/88	10/88-3/89	4/88-3/89
Psychiatrists	10	7	17
CPNs	1	1	2
Psychologists	0	1	1
Social workers	1	3	4
OTs	1	1	2
Vinten House staff	5	5	10
Not recorded	1	0	1
Sub-total	19	18	37
Not applicable	147	151	298
Total	166	169	335

There is also some indication that non-medical team members were responding on behalf of the service both more frequently and with increasing acceptability. In addition, immediate responses were increasingly being made both at the residential facility (still based on the main hospital site during the relevant time period) and at the new community base.

Response to referrals following team discussion A more even spread of response among the various professional groups within the team is indicated when we consider action following discussion in a weekly referral meeting, as shown in Table 4.18. There were also some interesting trends over time during the period studied.

Let us first consider the period April/September 1988. The staff at Vinten House and the team of CPNs respectively took action in respect of 29 per cent and 23 per cent of referrals, compared with the various psychiatrists doing so in 25 per cent of these instances. Social workers, psychologists and OTs also featured rather more prominently after team discussion than before. Recalling the figures reported earlier (Table 4.2) for the initial allocation of work during the preceding nine-month period, the respective proportions of new referrals taken up by Vinten House staff, CPNs and doctors then were 19, 32 and 29 per cent. Thus Vinten staff had already considerably extended their new work with clients in the community by the end of the first of the two six-month periods studied in more detail.

Turning to the period October 1988/March 1989, Vinten House staff and the team of CPNs respectively took action following team discussion in relation to 33 per cent and 21 per cent of the relevant new referrals, and the various psychiatrists in 23 per cent of these instances. The main changes between the two six-month periods analyzed in detail, regarding who took action following a team discussion, are therefore a further rise in the involvement of Vinten House staff and the appearance of joint assessments carried out by a CPN and the psychologist.

Table 4.18
Actors making initial response to referral after team meeting

	4/88-9/88	10/88-3/89	4/88-3/89
Psychiatrists	37	35	72
CPNs	34	31	65
Psychologists	8	8	16
Social workers	18	18	36
OTs	5	1	6
Vinten House staff	42	50	92
Joint assessment (CPN/psychologist)	0	8	8
Other	1	0	1
Not recorded	2	0	2
Sub-total	147	151	298
Not applicable	19	18	37
Total	166	169	335

This joint work was part of the establishment of a cognitive therapy group; where it appeared to the team that a newly-referred person might benefit from membership, assessment with this in mind was the next step. There was also a fall during this second period in the proportion of cases in which CPNs 'alone' made the initial direct contact with a new referral. The trends referred to were each most marked in the period from January to March 1989 inclusive. In part no doubt this reflects the development of the Cosham Continuing Care Group from late January and associated with this a period during which the CPNs who became part of the CCCG negotiated a reduction in their work with new referrals. There was also a drop in the OT's involvement with new referrals, due to her becoming the team's first formally-designated Co-ordinator.

In two cases concerning action following team discussion the actor was not recorded, but was probably in effect a member of the administrative staff acting on behalf of a duty officer or a member of the medical staff.

(There was one similar situation concerning action prior to a meeting - see Table 4.17). In each of these three cases, the action taken was a transfer or onward referral of one sort or another: one to a neighbouring area mental health team, one to the District Alcohol Unit, and a third to a psychosexual clinic. The single referral coded 'other' in Table 4.18 involved a decision to await the outcome of a court case which was pending.

Action taken following team discussion

The action taken as a matter of urgency in response to certain referrals (see Table 4.16) has already been discussed. In Table 4.19, which summarizes action decided upon after consideration at a team meeting, as a means of contacting the client for further assessment and discussion of possible ways of helping, we have used the various possible locations selected as most appropriate for further assessment as a form of proxy for the initial offer of help. The normal practice was to write to the client offering to visit or inviting them to come to one of the various possible venues. The initial assessment by the team may have identified a specific intervention as most likely to be appropriate; this would be reviewed and explored with the client when contact was made.

Table 4.19
Initial action taken after team meeting

	4/88-9/88	10/88-3/89	4/88-3/89
Domiciliary visit by consultant	1	1	2
Offered home visit by another team mber	47	54	101
Offered outpatient appointment	35	34	69
Offered contact at Vinten House	32	21	53
Offered contact at Acorn Lodge	n/a	23	23
Offered contact at a health centre	20	8	28
Transfer/onward referral	3	0	3
Other	5	9	14
Nothing recorded	4	1	5
Sub-total	147	151	298
Not applicable	19	18	37
Total	166	169	355

The pattern of the initial action taken after team discussion (Table 4.19) is best considered along with the information already given (Table 4.18) concerning who was primarily responsible for it. Considering first the period April/September 1988, a visit to the client at home by a non-medical team member - i.e. a CPN, a member of the Vinten House staff, or a social worker, psychologist or OT - was the most common offer, made in response to forty-seven (32%) of the relevant referrals. An offer of an outpatient appointment with one of the three medical members of the team was the second most common initial course of action following team discussion, occurring in thirty-five instances (24%). Our analysis of case files indicated that a significant proportion of these further assessments by medical staff led to the cases being quickly brought back to the team for further discussion, followed by reallocation to and action by a non-medical team member. An appointment at Vinten House was offered in response to thirty-two referrals (22%) and at a health centre in twenty cases (14%), after discussion at the referral meeting. The former usually involved Vinten staff, although these team members frequently also proposed home visits, especially where there was clear evidence of agoraphobic or similar tendencies. Offers of health centre appointments were usually made by the psychologists or by one CPN who, other things being equal, seemed to prefer this to a home visit. The social workers usually offered a home visit or, on occasion, contact at one of the other possible venues. This pattern and that from the logging data for the same period, presented in Chapter 2, are mutually confirmatory.

Turning to the period October 1988/March 1989, an offer of a home visit by a non-medical team member remained the most common response, occurring in fifty-four instances (35%): a slight increase. Offers of outpatient appointments remained the second most frequent response, made in thirty-four instances: approximately the same proportion as before (23%). The most striking change was in the use of Acorn Lodge as a location at which to see clients, following the partial move there in October 1988. This shift was most marked in the final three months of the period analyzed, during which the proportion of responses involving an offer of a home visit by a team member correspondingly declined. The use of Acorn Lodge also clearly took place at the expense of using health centres (most commonly used by team psychologists over the whole period). The new community base was the venue for the group of joint assessments carried out by a CPN and the psychologist, to which we drew attention earlier.

There was also a decline (from 22% to 14%) in the second six-month period in the use of Vinten House as a location for making contact with clients. However, Vinten staff also began to use Acorn Lodge for client contact before they themselves were based there. We noted earlier the increasing prominence of the staff of the residential unit in responding to new referrals. In addition to all twenty-one of the offers of contact at Vinten and eight offers of a home visit involving them, roughly half (11) of the twenty-three responses coded as 'offered contact at Acorn Lodge' in Table 4.19 involved staff of the residential unit. Once again, this evidence of changing patterns is mutually confirmatory with data produced by the (second) logging exercise (Chapter 2).

Included in the 'other' category for the first period in Table 4.19 are two invitations by Vinten House staff for clients to contact them (i.e. not specific offers of appointment), one instance of administrative liaison with the modecate clinic, one decision to await the outcome of a court case, and one situation where the client concerned died of a heart attack shortly after referral. For the second period, the 'other' category contains seven offers of an appointment for assessment but with no record of a specific location, and two invitations to make telephone contact.

Making contact with clients

We offer no detailed examination here of precisely what help was offered to clients, by what process of negotiation, and with what take-up and outcome. Some attention is given to these matters in Chapter 5, in respect of our interview sample of clients. However, our review of the case-files of all those people newly referred between April 1988 and March 1989 yielded some evidence as to whether the initial action taken by a member of the team following referral led to direct contact being made with the client concerned. Tables 4.20.1 and 4.20.2 summarize our findings on this point.

Direct client contact was made in 122 (76%) of the 160 cases where this was appropriate during the period April/September 1988 and in 139 (83%) of the 167 instances in which it was appropriate in the subsequent six months, whether urgently or following discussion at a team referral meeting.

Table 4.20.1
Making contact with clients in advance of team meeting

Outcome of attempted contact	4/88-9/88	10/88-3/89	4/88-3/89
Made as offered	17	16	33
Date/time changed	0	0	0
Venue changed	0	0	0
Contact after repeated offer(s)	0	1	1
No contact made	1	0	1
Nothing recorded re contact	0	0	0
Administrative action only	1	1	2
Sub-total	19	18	37
Not applicable	147	151	298
Total	166	169	355

Looking first at those new referral situations where action was taken prior to a team discussion, Table 4.20.1 shows that team members' attempts to make direct client contact were successful in all but one of the thirty-five relevant instances during the whole twelve-month period April 1988/March 1989. In two further cases the action involved was simply onward referral to another professional team.

Turning to attempts to make direct contact with clients following a team discussion, Table 4.20.2 shows that in respect of the 298 new referrals concerned during the period April 1988/March 1989, there was an attempt to make direct contact on the part of a team member in 292 instances, and that this was successful in 227 of them. 105 of these successful contacts took place during the period April/September 1988, representing 74 per cent of the 142 cases during that time where it appeared that direct contact had been sought following a team discussion. The corresponding figure for the period October 1988/March 1989 was 122, 81 per cent of the 150 relevant new referrals concerned.

Table 4.20.2
Making contact with clients after team meeting

Outcome of attempted contact	4/88-9/88	10/88-3/89	4/88-3/89
Made as offered	92	115	207
Date/time changed	6	2	8
Venue changed	2	1	3
Date and venue changed	0	2	2
Contact after repeated offer(s)	5	2	7
No contact made	30	23	53
Nothing recorded re contact	7	5	12
Administrative action only	5	1	6
Sub-total	147	151	298
Not applicable	19	18	37
Total	166	169	355

Thus, taking the twelve months as a whole, in 207 cases a single proposal to meet, made by a team member after discussion at a referral meeting, apparently led to direct contact with the client concerned on the day and at the time and venue proposed. Comparing the two six-month periods analyzed, there was a rise in the frequency with which this occurred, from 65 per cent (92 of 142) to 77 per cent (115 of 150) respectively of the referrals in each period where direct contact was sought following team discussion. In thirteen further cases the offered date, time or (perhaps more significantly) the proposed venue for meeting was changed in response to a request from the client. In seven cases a repeated offer, following non-response, led to contact being made.

In six cases, the appropriate response following team discussion was not for a team member to seek direct contact with the client concerned. Five of these were during the first period; four involved simply a transfer, onward referral, administrative check, or awaiting the outcome of a court case, whilst in one case the person referred died. In the second period, one newly-referred person moved away from the area before proper contact could be made.

In extracting information from case-files, an impression was gained that in a number of instances of referral during the period January 1989 onwards, the time elapsing between an offer and its take-up was longer than usual, without any record of more than one attempt at contact having been made. There were also some examples of longer delays between referral and team discussion than had been the case earlier. This could reflect the impact of an increasing workload, particularly perhaps the development of work with continuing care clients.

We examined our data a little further concerning the group of people newly referred during the two periods (30 and 23 respectively) where no contact had been recorded following discussion and decision at a team meeting. For the first period, the most striking feature of this sub-group as compared with the overall sample of new referrals was that a disproportionate number had been offered an appointment at Vinten House. There seemed to be a higher likelihood of a client not responding to an offer of an appointment at Vinten than of a home visit or a health centre or outpatient appointment. Although, as we saw earlier, there was a fall in the number and proportion of people newly referred in the second period who were offered contact at Vinten, this tendency persisted.

Home visits represented the most common form of post-meeting action throughout the twelve-month period analyzed, and also had among the lowest 'refusal rates', only failing to yield contact in two out of fifty-four instances. Offers of health centre appointments (much less commonly offered during the second period) and outpatient appointments also had relatively high take-up rates, with eight offers and no refusals and thirty-four offers and five refusals respectively. Offers of an appointment at Acorn Lodge during the period following the partial move there failed to lead to direct contact with clients in five cases out of twenty-three.

Whilst considerable caution is demanded in interpreting this material, it appears that during the year studied initial offers of home visits were more likely to be found acceptable by clients than were invitations to meet team members elsewhere, although outpatient or health centre appointments were much less likely to be rejected than were invitations to come to Vinten House or, in its first few months, to Acorn Lodge. A possible factor could be the staff involved; psychiatrists or psychologists were usually the team members seeing people as outpatients or at health centres, although appointments with nurses or social workers were rarely resisted when clients' homes were the suggested venue, regardless of which team member sought contact.

People previously known to the service made up a higher proportion of the sub-group where contact was sought following team discussion but where it appeared that no contact had been made, than did people previously known as a proportion of the total group of new referrals. Two further, but less marked, tendencies amongst the group of people apparently not contacted, also both persisting throughout the full year studied in detail, were a more even sex balance and a greater proportion among the younger age groups in comparison with the overall sample of referrals. Thus there is a suggestion that people previously known to the service, men, and younger people might be the most likely to resist offers of help, initially at least.

Summary

This chapter has offered an analysis of the referral process operating during the phase of our research prior to the move of the non-residential part of the Cosham service to its base in the local community and the period immediately following this partial move. We have examined certain characteristics of the people referred to the service from the community during the year from April 1988 to March 1989, splitting this into two six-month periods, one 'either side' of the partial move of the service in October 1988. Most of the data were drawn from 'the referral book' maintained by the team's administrative staff and from clients' case-files. Detailed attention to the two six-month samples of new referrals followed a preliminary analysis of new referrals during the preceding nine months.

Throughout the period studied in detail, the pattern of new referrals seemed to be relatively stable at some twenty-five to thirty per month, with some seasonal fluctuation. Twice as many women as men were referred, and two-thirds of the people concerned were not previously known to the service. GPs were overwhelmingly the main source of these referrals throughout, although there was a slight broadening in the range of professionals referring during the second six months of detailed analysis. There was very little evidence of clients themselves actively seeking help from the service on their own initiative, although this was slowly beginning to appear in the later stages of the year studied in more detail, with a very slight increase in self- and family referrals and a very small number of 'drop-ins'.

We have addressed the important but conceptually problematic question of the reasons for referral to the Cosham team, via a content analysis of the recorded statements of GPs and other referrers. Anxiety and/or depression figured predominantly as identified forms of distress for which specialist help was sought on these clients' behalf, with background difficulties in the areas of relationships and life events noted as significant contributors to these conditions. We also noted a trend away from requests for formal psychiatric assessment, perhaps indicative of changing expectations of the service on the part of referring GPs.

In a little over 10 per cent of referrals an urgent response was made, and in nearly half of these cases the action was taken by a medical team member. However, in the vast majority of referrals an initial team discussion first took place, with one member then identified as the person to seek direct contact with the client to further assess and negotiate the most appropriate and acceptable form of help. These referral/allocation meetings also discussed some of the cases already dealt with urgently, as well as certain other cases variously brought or referred back for further consideration by the team.

Initial response to referral, particularly following team discussion, was increasingly shared among all members of the team. We were able to indicate in our interim report (Powell and Lovelock, 1989a), when only the first of the two six-month referral samples had been studied, that the Cosham Mental Health Service was no longer one whose standard response was a domiciliary visit by the consultant or an outpatient appointment with a psychiatrist in a less urgent situation. This trend continued during the next phase of our study and, in addition, the staff of the inpatient unit serving the Cosham area increasingly became involved in working with newly-referred clients in the community, in addition to their residential commitments. This prominence took a further upward turn in the latter part of the year whose new referrals were analyzed in detail. During this period Vinten House staff, although still based on the main hospital site, were seeing clients at Acorn Lodge, the new base in the local community. The further increase in their involvement in part reflected the establishment of the Cosham Continuing Care Group and the heavy commitment of several team members, predominantly CPNs, to this work.

Where direct contact was sought with clients following discussion at a team referral meeting, it was successfully made in almost 75 per cent of cases in the first six-month period analyzed, rising to over 80 per cent in the six months following the partial move. Throughout the year studied, the most common approach to making direct contact with a client was a written offer from a non-medical member of the team to visit them at home. These offers, together with invitations to meet at health centres and outpatient appointments with medical staff, were more likely to result in take-up than invitations to come to Vinten House, on the main hospital site. Trends during the second period studied suggest that invitations by non-medical staff to Acorn Lodge, at least at first, were also less likely to lead to contact than home visits on their part or appointments with a psychiatrist or psychologist. The establishment of the whole service on the Cosham site, subsequent to the period for which we analyzed referral data, and further development of the team approach, may have altered these patterns.

A number of points emerge from the study of the referral process, particularly the analysis of new referrals over a one-year period, as reported in this chapter. Firstly, there is clear evidence of the increasing involvement of the residentially-based members of the staff team in responding to new referrals from the community, coupled with the impact on the work of the team as a whole of the development of the Cosham Continuing Care Group. These trends confirm the evidence of our logging study, presented in Chapter 2, and illuminate further the discussions which took place in team business meetings, reported in Chapter 1. Secondly, there is some evidence, based on recorded information concerning attempts to make direct contact with clients following discussion in a team referral meeting, that some locations were more acceptable than others to service users.

Finally and perhaps most importantly, this study of the referral process reveals the overwhelming predominance of GPs as referrers, and the extent to which 'anxiety and/or depression' was the main reason for them seeking specialist help on behalf of clients. By comparison, almost half of the referrals to the local social services area centre which had a mental health component were made by the person concerned her/himself or by a relative, and a significant number of referrals, particularly among this sub-group, involved practical problems or requests for practical resources (Chapter 3).

Such findings raise questions about what constitutes an appropriate referral to the specialist mental health service, and in turn about the nature, priorities and boundaries of the service as a whole. In the next chapter we explore these and other issues, drawing on the views of service users and of the main referrers to the Cosham team.

5 Service users

Introduction

We begin this chapter with an examination of the specific services offered, their take-up and outcome in a small number of situations. This is followed by a more detailed look at the process by which referrals for help were made, the nature of the service during the period of our study, and the impact of these various forms of help, through the eyes of the several different users of the service. The views of some of the people referred for help and of their relatives will be presented. These perspectives will then be complemented by the views of the professional workers who referred to the service: users in another sense. In addition to offering their views on a small number of particular situations, these users - appropriately all GPs in our sample - provided a wider professional perspective on the service as a whole.

Patterns of service use

Selection and characteristics of sample

To explore in some detail the pattern of services offered and used, a sample of new referrals was drawn from referrals made to the service during the six-month period October 1988 to March 1989: part of the partial move phase of the development of the service, in the terms defined earlier. This approach took account both of our limited time and resources and of the fact that some data had already been collected on new referrals to the service during the twelve-month period April 1988 to March 1989. The sample was constructed on the basis of taking every seventh referral made during the defined six-month period, thereby taking account of variations in referral rates over time. The total number of clients in the sample was twenty-three: 14 per cent of the 169 new referrals made during the period from which the sample was drawn. Table 5.1 shows the age and sex breakdown of the individuals involved.

Table 5.1
Age and sex of sample of new referrals (10/88 - 3/89)

Age	Male	Female	Total
under 20	0	1	1
20-29	0	4	4
30-39	2	6	8
40-49	1	4	5
50-59	2	2	4
60 & over	0	1	1
Total	5	18	23

Of the twenty-three clients comprising the sample, five were male and eighteen were female, an 'over-representation' of women in relation to the overall group from which the sample was drawn. However, the sample group included a number of people who had made significant use of the service over time (see Table 5.4); without this there would have been little point proceeding. Whilst there was a wider age range amongst the women included in the sample, there was a concentration of both men and women in the middle age categories, as in the overall group of referrals.

Table 5.2
Reason for referral

Anxiety and/or depression	16
Panic attacks	5
Life events	3
Relationship difficulties	4
Eating disorders	1
Total (mentions)	29

All of the referrals in the sample were made by GPs. The reasons for referral, taken mainly from GP letters, are set out in Table 5.2. Anxiety, depression, and frequently both in combination as 'anxious and depressed', were most commonly recorded, being mentioned sixteen times. In five situations there was a specific reference to 'panic attacks'. The reasons given for the referrals in the sample group fall into a broadly similar pattern to that for the whole group of new referrals over the same period, reported in Chapter 4, both in terms of stated sources or causes of distress and symptoms. As was that earlier discussion, the present table is based on items mentioned in the letters or other recorded reasons for referral; it therefore sums to more than the number of individual clients involved.

Services offered and used

Of the twenty-three people included in this sample, three were seen in advance of discussion at the regular weekly referral/allocation meeting. Two people, Mrs A and Mrs C (see Table 5.4), were visited at home by the consultant psychiatrist following requests from the GPs concerned. One person, Mrs F, was initially seen at home by the duty officer, a CPN, following a telephone call from her GP. The remainder, a substantial majority of those referred, were contacted following a team discussion. Table 5.3 summarizes the action taken following referral as a means of contacting the client for assessment and discussion of possible ways of helping. In all but one situation - one of those where an appointment at Acorn Lodge was offered - direct contact was established and an assessment made.

In addition to the two people already noted as seen at home by the consultant, seven more were initially seen by a member of the medical staff at an outpatient clinic. (All nine of these are marked with an asterisk (*) in Table 5.4.) A further seven people were seen at home by a member of the community team: five by a CPN and two by a social worker. Four people were seen by members of the residential team: three at Acorn Lodge and one at Vinten House. Two people were seen jointly by a clinical psychologist and a CPN: one at a local health centre and one at Acorn Lodge.

Table 5.3
Initial response to referral

Domiciliary visit by consultant	2
Offered outpatient appointment	7
Offered home visit by team member	7
Offered contact at Acorn Lodge	5 (4 seen)
Offered contact at Vinten House	1
Offered contact at a health centre	1
Total	23 (22 seen)

When direct contact was made, an offer of further help was discussed and accepted in the majority of cases. Table 5.4 sets out in detail the services offered to and subsequently used by the people in our sample, following initial assessment. Some indication of outcome is given, up to the point when data were collected, which in each case was at least six months after the referral concerned. In describing the type of service offered, the Körner codes for key activities have been used wherever possible.

Table 5.4
Patterns of service use

ID	Sex	Ivwd?[a]		Services offered/used	Outcome
A	f	m	*[b]	counselling (Vinten House)	moved away
B	f	i		counselling (home visits)	improved/case closed
C	f	r	*	ongoing assessment (home visits)	client ended contact
D	m	i	*	outpatient appointments	on-going
E	f	i	*	mutually agreed no further contact	
F	f	i		anxiety management/counselling (home visits)	improved/case closed
G	f	r	*	mutually agreed no further contact	
H	f	i		counselling (Acorn Lodge)	improved/case closed
I	f	i	*	cognitive therapy group (Acorn Lodge)	improved/case closed
J	f	i		counselling (health centre)	refused help
K	m	i		anxiety management/cognitive approaches/nlp[c] (home visits)	on-going
L	f	i		cognitive therapy group	refused
				counselling (several locations), relaxation group	improved/case closed
M	m	i	*	counselling (health centre)	on-going
N	m	m	*	referred to Drug Services	moved away
O	f	m		did not make initial contact	moved away
P	f	i		anxiety management/nlp[c] (home visits)	improved/case closed
Q	f	i	*	outpatient appointments, anxiety management/counselling (home visits)	improved/case closed
R	m	i		cognitive therapy group (Acorn Lodge)	improved/case closed
S	f	i		counselling (home visits)	improved/case closed
T	f	i		assessment (Acorn Lodge)	client ended contact
U	f	i		anxiety management (home visits)	ceased
				stress management course (Acorn Lodge)	ceased
				relaxation group (community centre)	on-going
V	f	i		counselling (home visits)	on-going
				relaxation group	refused
				inpatient episode	
W	f	i		counselling (Acorn Lodge)	improved/case closed

[a] In 3rd column: i=interviewed r=refused m=moved away
[b] * indicates initial contact with a psychiatrist
[c] nlp=neuro-linguistic programming

In the three situations where contact did not continue beyond initial assessment, the people concerned had all been seen as outpatients by medical team members. One was referred to local services for drug misusers; two terminated their contact with the mental health service by mutual agreement.

One-to-one counselling, frequently combined with anxiety management, figured most prominently among the forms of help offered, although the proposed location varied. Once initial contact had been established, few changes in venue occurred in individual situations.

More generally, where initial contact had been made by a team member other than a doctor, continuity of both team member and location was generally maintained. For example, all the users in our sample who had initially been offered a domiciliary assessment were subsequently offered ongoing contact in the form of 'anxiety management and/or counselling' at home. Of the four respondents initially seen at Acorn Lodge, all continued to be seen there for one-to-one counselling sessions.

Of the six users who had been seen initially by a doctor and who had further contact after this assessment, two continued to have regular outpatient appointments. In one of these cases, home visits from a CPN were also offered and accepted. One person was referred to the cognitive therapy group and another to the clinical psychologist for further assessment. Two people were offered ongoing assessment/counselling with a member of the residential team, one at Vinten House and one at home. In the latter case the client later terminated contact.

Two other respondents were also offered attendance at the cognitive therapy group, following a joint assessment by the clinical psychologist and a CPN.

In a small number of situations (4), more than one type of service was offered, either in combination or serially. In one of these cases group therapy or one-to-one counselling was offered; the latter was accepted. Given the reasons for referral in this sample, it is not surprising that counselling in one guise or another should be the most frequently offered form of help. However, as we observed in relation to the findings from our logging studies (Chapter 2), the choice of location and method of intervention may to some extent have reflected preferred personal styles of working amongst the staff team.

Users' views - clients and relatives

Interview sample and interviewing method

To gain a fuller understanding of these patterns of service use, and in particular a clearer indication of the impact of the various specific forms of help offered and used, we sought to explore the particular situations included in our sample more fully, primarily through the eyes of the individual service users and their relatives. In fifteen cases it was possible to identify a relative living at home: twelve spouses (including one cohabitee), two sisters and a parent. Thus our interview sample comprised twenty-three direct users and fifteen close relatives.

Eighteen clients out of the possible twenty-three were actually interviewed (see Table 5.4, 3rd column). Three had moved away from the district and could not be contacted. A further two, including one who was ill at the time, refused, both on their own behalf and that of their relative: a spouse (husband) and a sister.

Nine interviews were conducted with relatives: seven spouses (four husbands and three wives), a sister and a parent. There were four situations where the direct users agreed to being interviewed but refused our request to interview their spouse. Each of these instances was of a wife refusing permission for an interview with her husband. It was said both that these spouses had had no contact with the service, and that this lack of involvement was entirely appropriate.

The style of interview was considered very important and the approach used was similar to that employed in a number of our earlier studies (see Powell and Lovelock, 1987b). By adopting a conversational approach, respondents were encouraged to recount their experiences and views of the service in a relatively free and unprompted manner. To facilitate this process an interview schedule, rather than a structured questionnaire, was developed, to provide an overall framework for each interview. In this way it was possible to ensure that a broadly comparable range of issues was covered in every situation, whilst allowing for a degree of flexibility, within which the individual could feel free to express her/his views.

The main areas covered by the interview schedule were:

(i) the referral process - source of referral, reason for referral, and user's expectations of the service;

(ii) the nature of the services offered and used - initial contact, the elements of the service used over time;

(iii) the operation of the service, in terms of both its accessibility and its acceptability, its overall accountability, and its ability to provide a co-ordinated response over time;

(iv) the impact of the service on both the direct users and their relatives, in terms of its comprehensiveness and effectiveness, and their degree of overall satisfaction.

The interviews were audio taped and extensive notes, although not full transcripts, were subsequently prepared using the main topic areas of the interview schedule as a framework. The main issues explored in the interviews now provide a structure for analyzing the views of these users.

The referral process

Of the eighteen direct users interviewed, all had initially sought the help of their GP. The extent to which they had been encouraged to seek professional help varied considerably. One respondent had had a request for help mediated by his wife, who made an initial contact through a health visitor attached to the general practice. In several other instances a spouse, although not directly involved, had been very encouraging and supportive of their partner seeking help. In one situation a colleague at work had advised the respondent to seek help from her GP.

In making contact with their GPs the respondents had held varying expectations about the possible forms of help which might be offered. Three quarters of those interviewed had anticipated being offered medication. Of these, seven had specifically not wanted medication and were seeking an alternative, but unspecified, form of help. Six respondents had been prepared to accept medication, although in each case the GP had discussed alternatives. For example, Mrs L had expected to be offered medication, as she had been treated with tranquillizers in the past. However, her GP had suggested counselling, which she had thought a good idea as she felt she needed someone to whom she could talk. She recalled her feelings at the time:

> *You know, sometimes in my life I've felt as though I'm a bit topsy-turvy, because I'm very emotional you see. I suppose I went thinking that she'd stick me on tranquillizers to calm me down. I was very badly depressed and I felt I needed anti-depressants. I knew after a while they would pick me up, perhaps help me get over ... but then I still had a decision to make.*

In the majority of situations (two-thirds) the GP had initiated the possibility of a referral to the community mental health team. The extent to which these respondents had felt involved in the process of referral ranged from recalling only a very limited discussion to a sense of arriving at a joint decision. For example, one woman, Mrs U, who was suffering from severe panic attacks, had appreciated her GP's preparedness to discuss why he felt that this course of action might be helpful. She commented:

> *He suggested I saw a CPN, because they can explain to you how you're getting them [panic attacks] and what you can do to stop having them.*

Many respondents, like this woman, had been apprehensive about contact with mental health services. In such situations reassurance from their GP could be very helpful in allaying some of their uncertainties and, for some, their fears. Even the less apprehensive respondents had welcomed some explanation from their GP; several indicated their appreciation of having their difficulties taken seriously. Comments such as 'prepared to try anything', 'pleased to be offered some help', 'open to anything', 'surprised but prepared to try', were common.

Mirroring the varying extent to which these respondents had been involved in the referral process, were their feelings and expectations of the sort of help they might receive. Where the respondents themselves had initiated the possibility of a referral, they were not surprisingly rather clearer about wanting, as one respondent explained:

> *... somebody to talk to - they might tell me what to do about it.*

Even where there had been greater reluctance on the part of the respondent to seek help, there was frequently an acknowledgement of the desire to involve an 'outsider', with whom difficulties could be shared.

It is evident from these respondents' views that what was valued most was some acknowledgement of the need for outside help in resolving a personal difficulty. Whilst many respondents held particular views about the use of medication as a form of treatment, all seemed open to other suggestions made by their GPs and welcomed being involved in some discussion of possible alternative forms of help, including referral to the Cosham Mental Health Service.

Similar views on the value of an outsider were expressed by many of the relatives interviewed. In the few situations where a spouse had been actively involved in the referral process, the involvement of an outsider was especially welcomed. For example, in one situation where the spouse, Mrs K, had made the initial contact, she herself had wanted an opportunity to talk to someone outside the situation, as well as feeling this would be helpful for her husband. This perspective was shared by her husband, who in turn welcomed his wife's involvement in the referral process.

Services offered and used

All the direct users interviewed perceived the initial contact with a member of the team as some form of assessment of their difficulties, as well as an opportunity for a discussion of what forms of help might be available. Of the three respondents who were initially seen with a view to their attending the cognitive therapy group, one, Mr R, felt quite clear that the purpose of this initial contact had been to assess his suitability for the group. The other two respondents were less happy with what they perceived as a specific offer of help; they would have welcomed more discussion of other possible alternatives.

These perceptions raise issues both about the types of help offered and about the degree of choice available to individual clients. Being consulted about the sort of help you wanted and feeling involved in any decisions was much appreciated, even if the person concerned was fully prepared to follow the advice of the professional. Most respondents in fact felt that there had been sufficient discussion about the sort of help available.

In the few situations where this was not felt to have been the case, it appeared that ambivalence on the part of some clients may have prevented any attempt to open up the discussion. For example, Miss T had found the experience of individual counselling helpful as it had improved her self-confidence, but she had also felt that some form of group support might have been equally beneficial. She had not attempted to discuss this and had subsequently discontinued her contact. She had felt, as on many other occasions:

> *... intimidated by people in authority.*

Interestingly, her contact had been with a student nurse, and on a few occasions the nurse's supervisor had sat in on their sessions. This had not really worried Miss T, although she had sometimes felt that she was there, as she put it:

> *... more for the counsellor's training benefit [than for her own problem].*

Once again, she had not discussed this, as she had felt that the counsellor/student had been trying to help.

Of the two respondents, mentioned earlier, who initially had been reluctant to accept group therapy, one subsequently did so. The other, Mrs L, had more actively pursued one-to-one counselling, despite her feeling that the group was the staff's preferred option. As she explained:

> *[It was a] new thing and they were keen to get it off the ground, and I felt that I would have been a bit of a guinea pig.*

Acceptability

Our interviews indicated that some service users did not always feel sufficiently confident to initiate discussion about their needs. There can be a number of reasons for this; one important dimension of the issue is that of staff style, and in particular the ability of team members to respond in a sensitive and flexible way to each individual client.

Almost all the respondents found the staff with whom they had had contact very approachable. Words like 'friendly', 'sympathetic', 'welcoming' and 'helpful' were frequently used. An informal approach on the part of staff had been especially important in allaying many users' initial concerns. For example, Mrs P had received a letter from one of the CPNs, offering an appointment to visit her at home. At this first visit there had been a general discussion about her situation and how the service might be able to help. At the outset the woman concerned had been rather reluctant to seek help, but she had welcomed this contact in her home and felt reassured by the initial meeting, as she explained:

The fact that he explained to me there are a lot of other people with anxiety ... I was really - and probably still am really - ashamed of having had the problem. You know, it's something mental, it's something people don't talk about ...

The important part played by the friendly attitude of staff is also illustrated by this comment from another respondent, Miss S:

He's about my age, and I felt it was very, sort of, on a level: like a friendly chat and very, sort of, informal. I didn't feel intimidated in any way at any time. And again, that I can ask him when I want to see him rather than feeling that I had to see him.

All but two respondents would not hesitate to recommend the service to a friend, as the following comment made by Mrs W illustrates:

I didn't like it when people used to say to me: 'What are you going down there for?'; because I didn't tell people why I was going ... They think that they're totally crazy there, and I sort of try and explain to them it's not just for people that are mad or whatever ... There's everything down there; just people that can't cope; you know. I think it's a really good place.

Accessibility

The accessibility of the service in terms of location or venue was also seen as important by all those interviewed. All the respondents who had been seen at home were very appreciative of this type of contact. For example, Mrs L, who had been seen at several locations, had valued home visits:

The aspect of her coming to see you at home is dealing with you as a whole person, not just as an outside thing.

Relatives of spouses who had received home visits were also appreciative of this type of contact, recognizing that it was preferred by their spouse. Furthermore, it sometimes also gave them an opportunity to meet someone from the service and to feel more involved. A few relatives, for example Mrs K, expressed a wish for more contact or access to staff, although they recognized that this might lead to some difficulties:

I would like him [CPN] to have a session with me, either with or preferably without R [husband]. We say 'hello', but he'll never say anything to me about R, which I suppose is patient confidentiality, but he could ask me without giving anything away; but he never says anything and I think he should.

The slightly fewer respondents who had been seen at Acorn Lodge had also found this venue both easily accessible and acceptable. Given the choice, one respondent, Mrs W, had expressed a preference for contact at Acorn Lodge, as she explained:

> *I would rather go there because of the family being at home ... Actually I used to look forward to going down there, just to, sort of, talk about things.*

Relatives generally seemed less enthusiastic about contact away from the home, although their specific views varied. One spouse, who had had the opportunity to meet the clinical psychologist at a local health centre, where her husband was being seen regularly, would have much preferred having this contact at home. She had felt inhibited in an office setting and saw this as contributing to her not having found the session very helpful.

Another relative, a parent, would have appreciated some contact with the service. She had not had the opportunity to express this view, as her daughter regularly attended Acorn Lodge rather than having someone visit at home. Furthermore, Mrs T felt it would have been unfair on her daughter had she initiated any contact herself. As she explained:

> *I would have liked to have been involved to be quite honest ... because I could have put what I thought was my side of it too; it might have helped her. I was very tempted to, quite often, 'phone up ... Well I mean ... if she had a problem that was caused by us, I mean we have to admit our faults too ... I didn't feel the problem did stem from [parents' divorce], but you never know. I mean, children don't actually tell you those sorts of things, do they?*

Only one respondent expressed negative comments about a particular location; these referred to her initial visit to the residential unit, which at the time was still based on the main hospital site. Mrs J had found this venue quite difficult to reach by public transport, and on her arrival she had been uncertain of the exact location of Vinten House within the hospital grounds. Her first impression, coupled with the experience of being seen by a student nurse, albeit in the presence of his supervisor, unfortunately had not helped to make her initial contact a positive experience. This had led to her feeling unable to take up the offer of further help, although an alternative location, the Cosham Health Centre, had been suggested.

Quality of the service

The particular situation just referred to illustrates the complex interplay between accessibility and acceptability, and how together they form key features of any high quality service. These factors can substantially contribute to either a very negative feeling about the service, as suggested above, or an equally positive view, as the following example suggests.

Mrs H referred both to the building, in this case Acorn Lodge, and to the staff, as 'very pleasant'. She had felt fully involved in discussing a range of available options, and described the service as:

> *... a marvellous thing. I felt I fitted in with it.*

A similar view was expressed by a relative, whose wife, Mrs V, had had a brief stay in the residential unit. Mr V felt that both the location and the attitude of the staff were equally important. He was especially appreciative of his contact with the unit, summing up his experience thus:

> *What I liked about the place ... they made you feel welcome. I was very impressed with the staff; they were polite, very helpful. You could sit around and have a talk. The layout of the building ... the staff were very friendly. It was casual clothes, and they were very sociable. I thought it was really good.*

Co-ordination and accountability

Very few of the clients or relatives interviewed had any clear idea of how the overall mental health service was organized or how the different sorts of help fitted together. In the small number of cases where contact had been made either with more than one team member or at several different locations, the respondents held some notion of a team of workers based at Acorn Lodge. For example, Mr M mentioned that he did not understand why he had been seen in three different locations by three different members of staff, but he accepted - as did his wife - that it was usual to be passed from one arm of a service to another.

Only one respondent, Mrs U, had a relatively clear view of the overall service; this probably reflected her experience of receiving several different sorts of help. She described the service as offering a range of different forms of help, at home, at Acorn Lodge, and at other community locations. She explained her understanding of the service thus:

> *There are lots of different bits of treatment you can have, from what I can gather. I mean ... depending ... if you have a particular problem, let's use an example, say you're agoraphobic or something, you'd need counselling about how you can go out again on your own, build up your confidence. But then perhaps you were still a bit uneasy, you could go to some social activities, because they in some ways are just as important, because a lot of people I think get stuck between four walls for some reason or other. They seem to run a lot of things.*

No respondent had a firm idea of who might be in overall charge of the service, although one respondent, who had initially seen the consultant psychiatrist and then a CPN, suggested that the latter was:

> *... part of the doctor's team.*

Furthermore, there was considerable uncertainty over how any complaint or suggestion for improving the service could be made. Approximately half of the respondents said that, should it be necessary, they would get in contact with the staff member they knew at Acorn Lodge to discuss any difficulty. Slightly fewer said that they would discuss it with their GP. The remainder were uncertain of their likely course of action.

Comprehensiveness

A large majority of the respondents interviewed had had experience of only one aspect of help, generally in the form of one-to-one counselling. As a result, their assessment of the service tended to be focused around the significance of a particular form of help, rather than addressing the overall ability of the service to provide either a broadly-based or a comprehensive range of responses to meet a wide diversity of needs. One respondent, Miss S, commented on the lack of availability elsewhere of the counselling service that she had received:

> *I was very surprised that there was any service involved. I really did not expect anything and I feel very lucky to have had it actually: I really do. Because I know other people who've ... My cousin's had exactly the same thing as me and he's had no back-up whatsoever: nothing; not even from his GP: nothing. So I really do feel very fortunate.*

Only one respondent, Mrs U, referred to earlier as having been offered more than one form of help, had any appreciation of the diversity of the service. She had found her individual sessions with the CPN very helpful, as these had specifically addressed her individual problems at the time. The stress management course which she was subsequently offered had broadened her understanding and ability to cope with her anxiety. Her current attendance at a weekly relaxation class was presently meeting her need to maintain what she described as 'healthy living'. Furthermore, she felt that participating in a group activity was more beneficial than attempting to relax on your own at home, and explained this as follows:

> *[T]hey don't just help with your problem. There's lots of other things you can carry on and do; they broaden you out ... Acorn Lodge seem to run lots of little clubs and different things you can do.*

Impact of the service

Many of the respondents, in describing what difference being in contact with the service had made to them, used phrases like 'feeling more relaxed' or 'easing the tension'. Such feelings had often contributed to an increased sense of 'being able to cope' or 'help yourself'. One man, Mr K, summarized the views of several respondents when he commented thus:

> *I feel I'm calmer. I feel I know ... I suppose the first thing you know in a sense is that you're not the only pebble on the beach, you know. It's terribly easy to get very very inward-looking, so from that point of view it has been quite useful.*

He then went on to explain how this had enabled him to feel more able to cope with his situation and to help himself:

> *It's nice to have these people to talk to, and yes, they can help and suggest, but it really is you who's got to do something.*

This feeling of being enabled was shared by several respondents, as the following comment made by Miss S illustrates:

> *I think that probably the greatest thing was just to have somebody there if I needed them, who wasn't either a relative or a friend or whatever; who could give me a length of time which the doctor can't and who knew what he was talking about; sort of morale booster I saw it as really ... The problem I had, I had the help I needed. I really think it's something I've got to gradually overcome. I don't think anyone can really do anything about it as such, other than support me.*

This view was shared by her sister, who felt that she herself had also benefited from the help given to Miss S:

> *I think it's helped in that once she was told all about the condition, the anxiety condition that she's got, I think it helped her to come to terms with it more, and in retrospect how it had developed; and that helped us as well, because we didn't really understand, until she understood, what the problem was.*

Some respondents were able to be more specific about improvements either in themselves or their situations. For example, one woman, Mrs W, was no longer having nightmares, which was having a beneficial effect both on her and her family. In describing the difference that being in touch with the service had made to her life, she also conveyed something of the actual experience whereby she had been helped:

> *The nightmares were caused by some experience I had when I was younger. Going there, we just talked about basic things and I had to do a drawing and things, like a road of my life ... Going down there it helped me to accept it, because over the years, apparently, I must have blocked it out mentally, and it just came out in my dreams at night-times.*

Some relatives also spoke positively of noticeable signs of improvement, which in turn gave them a sense of relief and reassurance. One spouse, Mrs R, had been able to see some real change in her husband's behaviour, following his attendance at the group therapy sessions. She felt that he was now more able to assert himself and generally seemed more able to talk about anything that was worrying him. Furthermore, she felt that she had benefited from knowing that her husband was having professional treatment.

A sense of relief and/or reassurance that some outside help was being offered was, with one exception, shared by all the relatives interviewed. This one respondent, the spouse of Mr M, whilst seeing that it helped her husband to talk to an outsider, had not felt in any way relieved of her own worries and feelings of responsibility, despite having had some personal contact with the service herself.

Satisfaction

All but one respondent interviewed said they were either 'satisfied' or 'very satisfied' with the service offered to them or to their relative. Two respondents, Miss T and Ms I, whilst expressing some satisfaction with the help they had received, were critical about what they had experienced as a lack of choice. They shared the view that alternative forms of help other than those offered should have been more fully discussed. Furthermore, Ms I would have liked further contact with the service, preferably in the form of one-to-one counselling, when her group therapy ended:

> *Everyone was saying that [the group] was drawing to an end and we've had the support, and now suddenly it's like somebody's swiped the crutches from us.*

The dissatisfaction with the service expressed by one respondent, Mrs J, has already been touched on earlier in the text. She had experienced her contact with the service as a complete waste of time and had felt disinclined to take up the offer of more help. Furthermore, she said she had received little encouragement from her GP, whom she saw as having shown little interest in knowing about her contact with the service.

Many of the direct users of the service and their relatives whom we interviewed held overlapping or complementary views. However, this was not always the case. In a few situations there were differences in the levels of satisfaction expressed, with sometimes only a partial awareness on the part of a direct user of the benefits that being in contact with professional help could provide for relatives. For example, Mrs V had found it difficult to describe how the service had helped her, although she always looked forward to and enjoyed the weekly visits of the CPN. She was uncertain about the impact of the service, if any, upon her husband. He, however, described himself as 'very, very satisfied with the service'; knowing that his wife was receiving some professional help had also helped him. At one stage he had contemplated giving up his job, which involved working night shifts, because of his concern over his wife's condition. His worries had been considerably eased by the support being given to his wife and this had enabled him to continue in his present employment.

One recurring theme, evident from many of the users' comments about their feelings of satisfaction with the service, was a sense of personal achievement and a growing ability to help themselves. Mrs L spoke for many others when she commented:

> *They can offer you more help than you realize is going on. Well I saw myself as being cocooned within these four walls and not being able to get out. I think the part that she was from outside and she wasn't one of my friends, and the fact that it was an independent body really, who did not know anything about me, because family tend to get involved and take sides ... I suppose having someone's independent view ... I suppose she did help me to make that decision by helping me to think about myself. She made me look at it from a different point of view and made me feel I mattered ... She made me feel a person, after being everyone else's person. Now I'm me and I think for me and what I want.*

Summary

Overall, it was evident from the views of both the direct users and their relatives whom we interviewed that the service was seen as satisfactory. Families did not figure as prominently as direct users, but of those relatives interviewed, some sought closer contact with the staff from Acorn Lodge and others valued the support they had received and/or saw the service as having helped their family member.

Both the users' and their relatives' views and experiences highlight a number of important issues pertaining to the development of this and other would-be comprehensive locally-based services. Two key examples are: the complex interplay between the acceptability and the accessibility of the service in sustaining a person's commitment to stay in contact, and the sense of personal achievement and enablement, often associated with high levels of satisfaction, reported by several of those interviewed.

There was little evidence from these users of a wider knowledge or understanding of the service, beyond what they had experienced directly. Furthermore, beyond an unclear notion held by some that the doctor was in charge, respondents had little idea of how or to whom any concerns about the service might be expressed.

Whilst those interviewed had had varying expectations about the sort of response they would receive from their GP on first seeking help, each had appreciated some discussion of their situation, and the offer of either an alternative or an additional form of help to simply being prescribed medication.

It was evident from the users' views that GPs were seen as an important access point for help beyond the more immediate sources which might be available from families or friends. This role of the GP as the access point or gatekeeper to more specialist mental health services was one of the substantive areas explored in our interviews with GPs, reported in the following section.

Users' views - general practitioners

Introduction

The formal referral process operating during the twelve-month period April 1988 to March 1989 was discussed in Chapter 4. Throughout that period GPs were the main source of referrals to the Cosham service; our interview sample of referrers reflects this pattern. Referrers can be regarded as an important group of users of the service, albeit in a different sense from clients and relatives.

In each of the eighteen situations where a direct user of the service had been interviewed, the referring GP was identified. GPs were interviewed concerning a total of sixteen individual situations. In one instance the direct user had moved away and was no longer registered with the GP contacted; in another the GP was on extended leave during the period when the interviews were carried out. The number of actual GP interviews was nine. Five GPs were interviewed regarding one person and one concerning two of his patients, whilst three GPs were each interviewed regarding three situations. (The term 'patient', rather than 'client', is used in this section, to reflect more accurately the terminology used by the GPs interviewed.)

In addition to seeking the views of the GP concerned regarding each specific situation, the respondent's general views on the Cosham Mental Health Service were invited. The interview schedule described in the previous section, and employed with the direct users and their relatives, was also used as an overall framework for the GP interviews. Each interview was audio taped, apart from one where permission was refused, and transcribed in a similar way to that outlined for the other user interviews. Thus, as earlier, the main issues explored in the interviews also provide a structure for analyzing and presenting the GPs' views. Whilst the perceptions of this group of GPs cannot be taken as truly representative of all of the GPs using the Cosham service, they do provide a range of views and experiences of the service from the GP's point of view.

The referral process

Each of the GPs interviewed saw the referral process as involving negotiations, both with individual patients as potential users of the mental health service and with the Cosham Mental Health Team.

In the majority of situations it was the GP who had suggested the possibility of a referral, generally as an alternative to medication and/or as an opportunity to talk with someone able to offer greater time and expertise. This was explained by the GP who had referred Mrs W to the service:

> *I told her I didn't think she needed a psychiatrist, but it would help her considerably if she had a sympathetic person, who knew about such problems, to talk with ...: specialist support for chronic distress. She could understand this herself and that was why she was keen to go.*

Several GPs also found it useful to be able to refer a client when they felt that insufficient progress was being made. For example, in the case of Mrs L the GP commented:

> *If you're not winning with a degree of medical treatment ... I don't give tranquillizers: full stop ... I don't think she was keen either on taking anything else; that prompted the referral. She needed some degree of counselling and insight into her problems and the physical symptoms related to the anxiety, which I felt the CPNs could help her with.*

Another GP had used the service in a similar way, when he felt that Mr R had reached the stage of needing more specialist help. He explained:

> *I wanted some more expert help to try and sort out his depression, which I felt had been going on longer than I was prepared to accept without some progress.*

Several GPs commented on the changing expectations held by their patients about seeking help, and how these, coupled with their own desire to limit the use of medication, had contributed to a more extensive use of the service. They saw this as reinforced by the greater availability of counselling, as the following comment illustrates:

> *Patients have become much more aware of counselling services. More is written about it. More people are prepared to come forward and ask for help. We're using the service far more than we used to; well, it didn't used to be there. Looking back sixteen years ago in general practice, I think we used to throw drugs around, and we don't do that any more, so that we're looking at this ... as an alternative.*

In requesting help from the mental health service, all the GPs interviewed were conscious of being in a gate-keeping role. Some found this more problematic than others, depending on their own interests and commitments. As one GP commented:

> *[I've] noticed recently, over recent years, [the] last year or so, people will say: 'I want to see a counsellor'. That's very hard ... just to see yourself*

as a signpost doctor. I never say 'no', [but] sometimes I try and deflect it. I think that maybe they think we want to give them tablets, so in a way you can understand how they feel.

Another GP held a slightly different perspective on this issue:

It's a method of disposal when you've got a group of patients who are not physically ill. What channel do you direct them into for help? Even with an interest in this area you cannot take on this burden, so you have to find a way of dispersing them.

All the GPs interviewed confirmed that the majority of their referrals to the service were made by letter, and that they sought therein to convey something about the type of help they saw as necessary and appropriate. They were also aware of the weekly team meetings at which referrals were discussed and action decided upon. It was evident that a range of styles existed amongst the GPs interviewed in respect of referral letters. For example, one GP always wrote to the consultant, although often wishing to gain the help of another, non-medical team member. She explained:

Quite honestly now, I probably refer more through Dr [the consultant] to Acorn Lodge - and we do have to go through Dr ... of course - than I do to the psychiatrist [as such]. We are beginning to realize that a lot of people to whom we gave anti-depressants don't really need the anti-depressants, so much as the consistent counselling.

Another GP regularly addressed his letters to the team, although on occasions he would ask for a medical opinion:

I'm quite happy to refer to the team ... and they're prepared ... if I want something more specific, like a psychiatrist to see them ... they do that.

Some GPs had initially found it difficult to refer to the team rather than to a named individual, as this GP suggested:

We are used to referring to 'J. Bloggs'. I've got used to it now. Initially I found it quite hard referring to a team; it's easier to write to a named person ... Most of the time it has worked out. It's fine.

Another approach adopted by some GPs was to address the referral letter either to the team, when seeking a response to some psychological problem, or to the psychiatrist, when a specialist medical opinion was required. One GP was quite clear about what he intended to indicate by addressing his letters differently - although how far this was understood by the recipients remains uncertain. He explained:

In general terms, if it is an anxiety state or a phobia or panic reaction I would address it to the CPN. If it was a schizophrenic patient having major problems I would direct it to the consultant.

Thus the various ways in which these GPs sought help reflected their individual responses to the major change to an open referral system. It was evident that some GPs had more easily accepted the new system of making a referral to the team and had found satisfactory ways of getting the sort of help they wanted for the majority of their patients. This was summarized by one GP thus:

> *I'm gradually getting that feeling ... I think of them as a team, a fairly approachable team, in a different way to how I think of one of the consultant firms, with the hierarchy of staff and his secretaries and things; a group of people I know are there. And more recently, I have been able to rely upon them to take up the fight when my strength is weakening.*

Another GP held a somewhat similar view, and was prepared for the team to decide what course of action to take in any particular situation:

> *I don't object to the team looking at the referrals, because I think the doctor is not always the best person to sort out these things. Someone else may be far more appropriate.*

However, other GPs were less confident about the team's ability to make what in their own view was an appropriate decision, and tended to specify the type of help they wanted for their patient. One GP explained her reservations thus:

> *I do delegate that decision to the team, but I just feel a little uneasy that I don't know who the team comprises, and to whom I'm referring, basically.*

This view was shared to some extent by all the GPs in our sample in respect of situations which they identified as needing expert medical advice and ready access to the service's resources. They held very similar views about the sorts of situation where they wanted immediate access to a medical consultant, and were broadly in agreement that a request for a domiciliary visit was generally the most appropriate form of action. Their views and experiences seemed to vary, however, regarding the availability of a domiciliary visit by the consultant psychiatrist, as the following comments indicate:

> *If I had someone I thought was psychotic and needed admission, then I'd want a consultant straight away ... psychosis mainly ... If I think someone may need some heavyweight drug treatment, or maybe admitting, then I would tend to prefer a doctor to see them.*

> *I bypass the system by requesting a visit from the consultant ... at risk of suicide, floridly psychotic or severe depression requiring residential care ... perhaps someone to make a decision that: 'No; this person is not at risk'.*

I have very few patients who have a psychiatric illness or a psychotic illness; so I use it primarily as a counselling service. When we have a real psychiatric problem ... we're stuck and don't know what to do ... pray it won't happen ...

In these situations, where the GP was wanting an immediate response from the service, it was usual to make this request by telephone. For some GPs the availability of a duty system meant that they were prepared to consider, in some circumstances, other alternatives to a request for a home visit by the medical consultant; for example:

Anyone with a major psychiatric problem you would invariably suggest the psychiatrist, so that would be in the form of a domiciliary visit [and] tend to be acute rather than straight outpatient referral. If known to the service I might suggest a CPN assessment, and then they would speak to the consultant.

Other GPs were prepared to make more extensive use of the duty system, although the need to feel assured that someone was taking responsibility for the referral remained important:

I would ring up to speak to anybody I could get hold of: the duty officer. I'd want to give an immediate message. I wouldn't mind who it was given to, so long as someone was going to take action on it in the next forty-eight hours.

Some GPs found it useful to identify a named person and would then use this personal contact on subsequent occasions. One GP always tried to identify the named key worker, either directly from the patient or from any letter received, so that there was some channel of personal contact available if needed.

Generally the level of feedback received was seen as satisfactory, in as much as it was perceived as no different from that received from other parts of the hospital service. However, many of the comments made in this area do raise issues concerning the accessibility of the service to its referrers and the vexed question of accountability. Both are given further consideration later.

Nature of the services available

Although the GPs interviewed seemed to have relatively little detailed knowledge about the possible forms of help available from the Cosham Mental Health Team, they shared a general view of the service as one which had gradually expanded its counselling activities. As one GP suggested:

It deals with psychiatric diseases in the community and stress: severe stresses of life, where people can't cope. They try to help them get over that. Obviously the services were set up ... and even though they've got the background to deal with psychiatric illness ... they're probably spending most of their time dealing with the other.

Another GP was more specific in describing the sort of service she saw Acorn Lodge providing for most people she referred:

The availability of somebody to whom they can talk, who will try, with professional knowledge, to help them with their problems ... mostly emotional problems and attitude towards life or other people or to what's happened to them.

Although these quotations exemplify the main uses of the service reported by the GPs interviewed, they also sought its help with more formal psychiatric problems, as one GP explained when discussing Mrs Q's situation:

Slipping from a neurotic to a psychotic state of mind; fairly at risk living on her own, particularly in view of her age. I thought we ought to intervene to get someone more experienced than me to assess the severity of the mental illness.

Acceptability and accessibility

When commenting on the acceptability of the service, most GPs confirmed the views of the direct users, describing the staff as 'approachable'. However, they did raise issues concerning difficulties in sustaining contact with some patients, and how personal motivation was an important factor. For example, in confirming Mrs W's positive experience of the service, her GP commented:

She was obviously able to talk to the person she saw. She was a good patient to refer ... co-operative, who welcomed the help it would give her and her family. She didn't give up after one or two sessions.

Another GP made a similar, although more general comment concerning some people with more severe mental health problems:

With the more serious psychiatric illnesses, sometimes I've found follow-up discontinued, if the patient says: 'I don't want to see you any more'. Sometimes it coincides with a change in key-worker, or someone is away on holiday. Then the whole thing crops up again a month or so later, and because the person has relapsed it starts all over again. That's occasionally a bit of a breakdown in communication. If they had said to me: 'Should we discontinue or try to carry on?', we could have discussed it.

All the GPs saw the local service as offering a more acceptable form of help than had previously been made available at the main psychiatric hospital, some four to five miles away. It was seen as less stigmatizing for its users, as this GP's comment suggests:

> *... [m]ore approachable now. It's much easier to get at; far less stigma from the patient's point of view. They are much happier to go there than before ... A definite benefit.*

Another GP commented thus:

> *When we had to send them to St James' there was a great block; they didn't want to go. Now we just call it 'counselling round the corner', and they will accept it* [sic]. *They don't realize it's part of the mental health service.*

Some GPs, whilst acknowledging the benefits of a local service, did not see it as significant for those people requiring inpatient care. For example:

> *The softer psychiatry is more appropriately handled by having a local service. The more serious stuff ... I don't think it makes a lot of difference.*

One GP, however, had visited a resident at Acorn Lodge and found the setting less daunting than the psychiatric hospital, where he had also visited patients:

> *[It's] quite bright compared with the negative feelings I get about St James'. Acorn Lodge has a good feeling. The decor and the way they have got it is very reasonable.*

This particular GP liked to visit his patients 'in hospital', seeing this as a way of getting to know more about the service as well as maintaining contact with the resident. However, he had not found his initial visit entirely straightforward:

> *When I popped up to Acorn Lodge the door was locked, and when I tapped on the window someone came along, and they're not sure who you are - rightly so - but there is a bit more of a barrier to popping in to see how a patient is doing.*

Some GPs, although they had not visited the premises, nevertheless saw the service as an identifiable part of their local network. One GP commented:

> *[It's] more accessible from the point of view you can ring up Acorn Lodge and there is someone on call there. If you've got a problem, they'll deal with it straight away. There isn't anything to worry about. Ringing St James' used to be harder; there's no doubt about that.*

This view of a more accessible service was confirmed by another GP:

> *There is a limited number of people who you will be contacting, rather*

than a conglomerate at St James', which is obviously better.

However, this was not a view universally shared, as one GP who had found it necessary to refer to all three city teams commented:

> *Most teams have made an effort to get to know us. I just feel that the system, as it has become, is so fragmented ... although it seems to be working. But everybody feels it doesn't seem to be working as well as it used to.*

This GP had also had the experience in the past of having a clinical psychologist based at her surgery, and had appreciated the benefits of such an attachment. Not surprisingly, she felt that some positive elements of the service had been lost, and expressed a preference for it to:

> *... [go] back to what it used to be, all in one place, with ready availability. Similarly, I would very much like, in the surgery, a social worker allocated to us, or maybe a psychologist to do the assessments as she used to do.*

Although commenting positively on the service that both Mrs L and Miss T had received, this GP felt that things could have been handled rather better under the previous system:

> *... could have been discussed, counselled and dealt with in a fairly short space of time. The outcome would have no doubt been the same. It is not a question of quality; just availability and time.*

Accountability

The extent to which the service was seen as accessible to its referrers, in the sense of being readily available, was linked for some GPs with the question of accountability, about which some concern was expressed. The main issues were around team leadership and overall accountability for clinical matters.

Observations on the referral process, reported earlier, indicated that for some GPs the leadership issue was not an immediate concern, so long as there was a response and that access to medical support was both available and made use of as appropriate. Some of the GPs who took this view continued to refer to the medical consultant although seeking access to other team resources, for example by using such an approach as:

> *Could one of your team see this person?*

However, other GPs were less satisfied with this aspect of the service; whilst acknowledging that a referral to the team opened up a wider range of options, they felt that it could also lead to a lack of medical input and possible confusion as to who might hold overall medical responsibility. For these GPs the role of the consultant psychiatrist as someone with an overview of the situation was essential. For example:

> *When you're referring, they don't always go to a person who you know. There is no guarantee that the consultant will see them or have an overview of the patient.*

An inter-related concern, expressed by two GPs, was the involvement of student nurses in situations where specialist help had been requested. Whilst the need for this type of training for nurses was accepted - reluctantly in some cases - these GPs remained concerned about the need for adequate supervision and appropriate accountability over clinical matters.

Impact of the service on patients

Overall, the majority of referrals made by GPs were for counselling services. All the GPs interviewed were satisfied with this aspect of the help offered, both in general terms and more particularly in relation to the sample group. For example:

> *I think that I would say that as far as I'm concerned, those patients that I have referred, who have wanted to be helped by the service, have indeed been helped.*

Rather more specifically, another GP, in discussing the help that both Mrs U and Mrs F had received, felt that the service had been successful in providing them both with:

> *... insight, and showing them how to relax, giving them books and leaflets to read on symptoms that can arise from anxiety. They then have total understanding and then they look for ways, obviously, of trying to control their anxiety and panic attacks; and so it's a learning process. The CPN has far more time than we have ... Successful treatment and no further problems: not coming back a year later.*

All the GPs interviewed said that when referring they anticipated a suggestion of one-to-one counselling; they saw this as the most commonly offered form of help, although some were aware of a number of alternatives. As one GP commented:

> *He had group therapy ... [It] worked fairly well for Mr R; it worked out very well, but took a long time.*

The following quotations represent one GP's attempt to summarize the types of help available. He expressed a widely-shared overall view of the service:

> *It gives me a specifically trained and sympathetic group of paramedical staff, who are able to deal with the majority of psychological problems*

> *that walk into my surgery, but which I haven't got the time to deal with. Bearing in mind, having said that, that probably only one out of thirty or more that I see would I need to refer, because the rest I would manage to deal with some way, or they get better fairly quickly.*

He included Mrs B, whom he felt had benefited from her contact with the service, in this group. He continued:

> *The next category is for the more seriously ill psychiatric patient, who I feel I can probably diagnose fairly accurately but who is not responding to the level of medication that I'm prepared to give them as a GP, and who probably needs some support at home as well. Basically someone who I've been treating for a month or two, like Mr R, and I'm not making enough progress; a substantially smaller group.*

He concluded:

> *Out of ten referrals, six or seven would be in the first category, another two in the second category, and a very small fraction, less than one in ten, the very severe who possibly needed admission or a domiciliary visit ... The fact that it's the Cosham Service makes no difference; I need a psychiatric assessment and that would work just as well under the old system as the new one.*

Impact of the service on GPs

All the GPs interviewed saw the Cosham team as providing them with a service, and one which they were increasingly using, primarily for many of their patients wanting help with psychological difficulties. This was generally seen as relieving the GPs' ever-growing workload of this nature. For example:

> *Before Acorn Lodge, I would probably have dealt with them or tried to deal with them on my own, because I don't really think that it was for the psychiatrist to deal with. So I think I tried and spent many hours ... [It's been] a very great help actually.*

She continued:

> *Less emphasis on the psychiatrist ... A lot of work is done by not medically qualified, but well-qualified people; that alone has made a lot of difference. I refer more, but not to the psychiatrist.*

Another GP, acknowledging the impact on both the direct users - his patients - and himself as a 'professional user', confirmed this view:

> *Better than it was before; all round excellence. The CPN service has been very, very good indeed, and helpful. ... support, treatment and help to the patients, and then indirectly to doctors, because obviously one is*

concerned about one's patients. And if you haven't got the service the patients aren't getting better and therefore your workload is greater, because you're having to deal with problems or chronic problems. Therefore without the service we would be in trouble.

For some GPs this sense of being relieved was helpful, even if they knew that they would continue to be involved as the family doctor. As one GP explained:

Quite helpful from the point of view ... for me to take time out ... being at the coal face for a particular patient ... for someone else to take the burden for a little while.

Overlap between the services was generally seen as inevitable in some situations, as the GP frequently continued to have some contact with her/his patient, possibly to provide a medical certificate or for other 'unrelated' health problems. This could create some uncertainties, as this GP explained:

I never know quite how to play it once I've sent them to Acorn Lodge. If it's someone I've got quite involved with, I don't know whether to continue to be involved.

Another GP expressed a different view:

Once you've referred someone with a diagnosable or relatively clear-cut psychiatric illness, it's their pigeon until they've either got them fully better ... or if they want to involve the GP again, they do so on a formal basis. They don't just sort of forget about the patient, so they have to go back to the GP again.

The GP just quoted was essentially referring to people with longer-term mental health problems. Overall, however, the GPs interviewed seemed to have very little contact with this group, as one GP explained:

They are not often seen, because probably they know where to go and that's probably right.

Another GP was rather more cautious when making his response:

There's no real way of measuring. They're not bothering me. As this service is demand-led, I presume they're alright.

Work with people with longer-term mental health problems was not generally perceived as making high demands on GPs, nor was it seen as an immediately pressing concern by our sample group of doctors.

Fostering closer links

A range of views was expressed as to the appropriateness of establishing closer links between the two services: that provided by the GPs and the primary health care team, and that of the Cosham Mental Health Service. As we observed earlier, for some GPs simply having a named contact was sufficient; for others a more personal contact was highly valued, as suggested by the GP who had had the experience of working closely with a practice-based clinical psychologist.

Another GP had also had a clinical psychologist based in his practice, although this arrangement had ceased some considerable time ago. However, the practice had established and retained regular contact with a CPN: also a member of the Cosham team. The positive feature of this informal liaison, in the view of this GP and his colleagues, was the knowledge that a representative of the mental health team would be visiting the practice regularly, around twice a month, and at known times. Because this personal contact could be relied upon, many queries could be left for discussion on these occasions. Some feedback on patients previously referred, together with an opportunity to discuss potential referrals, represented the main focus of these visits, which were highly valued. This GP considered it important that the liaison person should have had some direct involvement with some of those clients referred by the practice, as well as some knowledge about how others were being dealt with by the team.

Two other GPs spoke of the potential advantages of having some form of attachment, which might foster closer working relationships between the two services. Both saw this as primarily a liaison role, similar to that described in the previous paragraph. However, one of them raised the possibility of actually locating a team member within the group practice surgery, but felt that such an initiative would receive a mixed response from fellow-GPs. On the general matter of such ways of working together she commented:

> *... [no] pat answers, otherwise it would have been done; different GPs, practices and populations.*

Another GP had a particular proposal for closer working links between the primary health care team and the Cosham service:

> *The only thing that I wish there were are some groups, post-natal groups, because there are lots of people I see who are sliding into post-natal depression. Perhaps a group would be useful. It could be a role for Acorn Lodge or the health visitor. There's a gap there and it's hard to bridge.*

Summary

These GPs' views of the referral process largely confirmed the views of their patients, the direct users of the service, that the majority of referrals were made as an alternative to medication and as an opportunity to talk with someone about areas of psychological distress.

The view of the GP as gatekeeper or access point to the Cosham service was also shared by these two groups of users. The GPs offered a range of views regarding the establishment of a system of open referral to the team. Many GPs accepted this system as opening up access to other resources, although for others it remained an area of concern. A small number of GPs took the view that overall responsibility should rest with the senior medical member of the team; others were less concerned about this particular issue, but did want immediate access to medical resources in situations which they perceived as requiring an urgent response.

The GPs' views of the service as being more acceptable and accessible, now that it was sited in the local community, mirrored those of the direct users and their relatives. Some GPs raised the issue of how a user's contact with the service might be better sustained, which was something also emerging in the views of the direct users.

Overall, the Cosham service was perceived by these GPs as providing an important source of help for their patients, primarily in the form of a counselling service, although by no means exclusively so. For themselves, the GPs saw the service as offering some relief from the increasing demands being made on their time and resources by patients seeking help with psychological difficulties. It also gave them access to specialist help and resources, and an opportunity to 'share the care' in some situations. As these GPs had little contact with people with longer-term mental health problems, they rarely made use of the service for this group of clients, unless presented with a 'crisis situation'.

Summary

In this chapter we have examined a number of key aspects of the developing community mental health service in Cosham via the views and experiences of its direct users, their relatives, and the GPs who, in the main, referred people for help to the team, and who are themselves users of the specialist service in a different sense. It is evident that from their various perspectives these groups had broadly similar and generally positive views about the nature and value of the service.

As we saw in Chapter 3, when exploring the development of continuing care services, users' views highlight key issues about the nature of the service and its priorities, and the 'negotiated boundaries' between the service and its major partners, in this case the GPs. In the next chapter we explore these areas further, focusing our attention on the perspectives of the front-line providers of the service and their changing roles within it.

6 Professional practice

Introduction

Service initiatives such as the decentralization of adult mental health care via multidisciplinary patch teams have far-reaching implications for professional practice. The successful development of community-based services demands that staff adopt very different roles from those appropriate to the hospital setting. Aspects of the changing nature of the various team members' roles and tasks have been evident throughout the previous chapters. In this short chapter we focus on the views held by members of the Cosham Mental Health Team as these changed and developed with experience over the period of our study.

Staff attitudes about the changing service

In order to explore the impact of the change of service-base from hospital to the local community from the service providers' perspective, we undertook a systematic examination of staff views on a number of key issues surrounding the development of 'care in the community'. The various findings presented in earlier chapters, drawing on different sources of information, have indicated the prominence of themes such as teamwork and the management of service priorities in the development of the Cosham service. To examine systematically team members' attitudes towards developing community-based services and working as part of a multidisciplinary team, we used a specially-designed self-complete questionnaire.

Our questionnaire contained a range of statements about the provision of services for people with mental health problems. Each team member was asked to consider the statements in turn and to place a tick under the column heading which most closely reflected her/his degree of agreement/disagreement. Four pairs of questions explored the potential advantages and disadvantages of teamwork. A further set of eight questions, again in pairs, examined certain common assumptions about community care, focusing around the possible patterns of service delivery and practice appropriate to the development of a community-based service. Three single statements referred to certain general issues, in particular aims and priorities regarding the direct provision of a specialist service, encouraging service development, and promoting user involvement.

The same questionnaire was used on two separate occasions: once just prior to the first stage of the move, and again five months after the whole service had come together on the same site. On the first occasion the questionnaire was completed by twenty-one team members: four CPNs, the senior OT and OT helper, the clinical psychologist, two social workers and the consultant psychiatrist, all then based at North Lodge, plus the Clinical Manager, nine nurse therapists and one clinical teacher/joint appointee then based at Vinten House. On the second occasion the questionnaire was completed by twenty team members: four CPNs, the senior OT and OT helper, two social workers, the clinical psychologist, the consultant psychiatrist and the clinical teacher/joint appointee, all based in the community office at Acorn Lodge, plus the Clinical Manager and eight nurse therapists based in the residential unit, also by this time forming part of the overall service at Acorn Lodge. (The Assistant Clinical Manager was on sick leave at the time of collecting this second set of data.)

The findings from these two exercises are presented together, in order to examine to what extent changes occurred as the service evolved and developed in the community. However, although the numbers of respondents in the two groups, and their general composition, are very similar, it must be remembered that there were a number of individual staff changes over the intervening period. Differences between the two reported sets of responses must therefore be treated with some caution. To encourage this, in discussing the detailed findings we generally refer to 'the first group' and 'the second group' of respondents, or to 'the first study' and 'the second study', rather than to 'the first occasion' and 'the second occasion'.

The nature of the service

A similar overall pattern of findings emerged from each set of responses, suggesting substantial team agreement over time regarding the nature of the service. There was broad agreement with the view that 'working together with non-professionals, volunteers and users of the service is essential to the development of a comprehensive mental health service'. Twenty-one respondents from the first group and nineteen respondents from the second group agreed with this statement. This included ten and nine respondents from the first and second studies respectively who strongly agreed. One respondent in the second study disagreed. There was also broad agreement with the statement that 'working to support other agencies ... in the care of people with mental health problems is as necessary as offering a direct service to clients'. Twenty respondents (five strongly) prior to the move and nineteen respondents (nine strongly) following the move agreed with this statement. One person in the first study disagreed, and one person in the second study was uncertain.

There was less overall team agreement with the view that 'our first priority must be to provide a specialist, treatment-orientated service to individuals and families'. Once again, however, this pattern remained the same over time; in both the first and the second groups fourteen respondents agreed with this view. Three (of the fourteen) strongly agreed, three were uncertain, and four disagreed in the first study, with this range of response spread across the whole team in terms of the various professions represented. In the subsequent study, one (of the fourteen) strongly agreed with this statement, two disagreed, two expressed uncertainty, and two respondents did not make their views clear.

Teamwork

There was overall general agreement from the respondents on both occasions that from the client's point of view teamwork was preferable to individual responses, and that teamwork provided a supportive rather than a restrictive working environment for staff members. Twenty respondents in the first study, and nineteen in the second, either agreed (11 and 9) or strongly agreed (9 and 10) with the statement that 'teamwork is better than individual work as a way of providing a client-centred service'. One person disagreed with this statement prior to the move; one expressed uncertainty following the move. This general agreement on the value of teamwork was confirmed by widely-shared disagreement with the statement that 'teamwork can easily lead to fragmentation of services and confusion for the users'. Fourteen people disagreed, one of them strongly, two were uncertain, and five agreed with the statement in the first instance. Subsequently, thirteen respondents disagreed, three were uncertain, and four agreed with the statement.

A majority of respondents on both occasions (19 and 16 respectively) disagreed with the statement that 'professional or clinical autonomy is severely restricted by team membership'. Two people in the first group agreed with this view, whilst in the second group three people agreed with the statement and one person was uncertain. In response to the statement that 'multidisciplinary teams provide staff with many opportunities for personal development and mutual support', fourteen people in the first study agreed and six strongly agreed; one disagreed. A broadly similar response was obtained from the second study, with seventeen respondents agreeing with the statement, six strongly, whilst two were uncertain and one disagreed.

There was less agreement overall in the responses regarding the decision-making process and the necessity for a blurring of roles. In the first study, seven respondents agreed, one strongly, with the statement that 'team members with particular expertise, experience or competence should play a more active part in team decision-making', three people were uncertain, and eleven disagreed, two of them strongly. Once again the range of response was spread across the whole team. A similar spread of views across the team was also evident in the second study, although the balance of views was reversed, with fourteen people agreeing, three strongly, with the statement, four respondents disagreeing, and two being uncertain.

There was a somewhat higher overall level of team agreement regarding the statement that 'all team members should have equal power and involvement in problem-solving and decision-making', although the responses over time were different. Prior to the move, fifteen members agreed with this statement, three strongly, one was uncertain, and five disagreed; after the move, six agreed with this statement, one strongly, one was uncertain, and thirteen disagreed, three strongly.

In response to the statement that 'successful teamwork is only achieved through the blurring of professional boundaries and an overlapping of roles', the range of views expressed was broadly similar over time. In the first study, nine respondents agreed with the statement, three were uncertain, and nine disagreed. At follow-up, seven agreed, two were uncertain, and eleven disagreed, two strongly. This range of views was also evident in the responses to the statement that 'a differentiation of roles and a clear division of labour promotes effective teamwork'. In the first study, eleven team members agreed with this statement, four were uncertain, and six disagreed, two strongly. In the follow-up study, twelve respondents agreed, three strongly, three were uncertain, four disagreed, one strongly, and one respondent's views were not known. As before, the range of responses was spread across the whole team.

Care in the community

There was widespread agreement with the statement that 'with modern approaches even people with severe mental health problems can live reasonably normal lives in the community'. Seventeen respondents in the first study agreed or strongly agreed (2) with this view, one was uncertain, and three disagreed, one strongly. These responses were consistent with those recorded in relation to the statement that 'people with longer-term needs are better off when they can live in hospital in peaceful surroundings'. Seventeen people disagreed with this statement, three strongly, three were uncertain, and one strongly agreed. A similar pattern of responses was evident from the second study: seventeen respondents agreed with the former statement, four strongly, one strongly disagreed, and two were uncertain; seventeen team members disagreed with the latter statement, three strongly, and three were uncertain.

The team's shared commitment to community care was similarly expressed in the responses to the statement that 'with adequate community services the need for residential care is minimal'. In the first study, seventeen people agreed with this statement, four strongly, one was uncertain, and three disagreed. There was equally strong agreement with the statement that 'there will always be a need for some form of hospital care ...'; here eighteen respondents agreed, five strongly, two were uncertain, and one strongly disagreed. These views were broadly consistent over time: at the follow-up stage, seventeen respondents agreed with the view that the need for residential care was minimal, seven strongly, one was uncertain, and two disagreed, one strongly. Nevertheless, an equal number of respondents (17), also agreed with the view that some form of hospital care should remain, three strongly, and three disagreed.

There was a substantial measure of agreement with the statement that 'traditional practices must be challenged and replaced by radical new approaches to caring ...'. Prior to the move, thirteen respondents agreed, four strongly, four were uncertain, and four disagreed. Following the move, fourteen agreed, one was uncertain, and five disagreed. However, only slightly fewer agreed with the statement that 'shifting services from the hospital ... is happening so quickly that we are discarding some good elements along with the bad or outdated'. Prior to the move, twelve people agreed with this statement, three strongly, three were uncertain, and six disagreed, with a similar pattern of responses - thirteen, one, two, and five respectively - after the move.

There was widespread agreement with the statement that 'the skills required to work effectively with clients are equally valid in work with other professional workers and informal carers in the community'. In the first study, nineteen team members agreed, eleven strongly, whilst two disagreed. Subsequently, seventeen respondents agreed, seven strongly, two were uncertain, and one disagreed. However, the team's views were rather more evenly balanced in response to the statement that 'working with other agencies and networks already established in the community requires a different sort of expertise from that required for direct work with clients'. Again a consistent picture was also evident over time.

Eleven people agreed with the statement prior to the move, two of them strongly, and ten disagreed, two strongly. Ten respondents agreed with this statement, two strongly, and ten disagreed, including one strongly, at follow-up.

Summarizing the findings from this study of staff attitudes over time, there appeared to be broad agreement within the team about the type of service to be provided. Both working together as part of a team and collaborating with other agencies and local networks were consistently seen as important activities in developing the service. Whilst there was general agreement that working as part of a team offered support and opportunities for professional development for staff and a better overall service for clients, there was less agreement about the actual processes involved in working as a team. This was particularly evident from the range of views expressed concerning decision-making and the extent to which individual team members should retain specialist skills or seek to acquire new ones. Furthermore, it was also in the area of decision-making that there was most evidence of change in the team's responses over time. Whereas in the first study there was a tendency to support the view that team members should have equal power in decision-making, this was reversed on balance in the second study, with a shift towards the view that team members with particular expertise or experience should be more active in this process.

Satisfying and dissatisfying aspects of work

In addition to indicating their degree of agreement/disagreement with our series of statements, each respondent was asked to identify the three most satisfying aspects of her/his work. Almost all the practitioners saw their direct work with clients as a satisfying dimension; this was the most consistently recorded comment over time. Where this was not specifically mentioned, a positive reference to being able to respond flexibly to a person's needs was reported. The second aspect of their work most commonly mentioned by respondents on both occasions as satisfying was being part of a team. This was seen as providing opportunities for joint working and mutual support. In addition, one feature of teamwork frequently recorded positively was an involvement in setting up special projects, participating in new groups, or initiating service developments generally. This was more evident in the second study, when slightly over half of the respondents specifically mentioned their service development activities, often in association with opportunities for working with other agencies, as a source of satisfaction. A range of comments about opportunities for professional development, professional autonomy, and the flexibility of roles and tasks, formed another substantial group of positive responses, as did teaching activities.

In a similar way, respondents were then asked to record the most dissatisfying aspects of their work. Time seen as spent unproductively, either in meetings or in form-filling, was the most frequently mentioned single area of dissatisfaction in the first study. This was confirmed in the later study, although it was less frequently commented upon than future uncertainty concerning the NHS generally. Several observations on this topic referred to likely changes in the organization of services and the availability of resources. A concern about the impact upon their day-to-day practice of wider changes in the provision of health and social care was also expressed by members of the team.

Many comments, on both occasions when the questionnaire was used, focused in a general way on a felt lack of support other than that experienced from colleagues within the team. This was sometimes expressed as a lack of support from management, coupled with a felt lack of awareness on the latter's part of the practitioner's experience, or as a general feeling of uncertainty and a lack of downward communication. References to a shortage of resources and insufficient time, linked with experiencing excessive demands, also made up a substantial group of comments. Poor communications within the team were also mentioned in the second study, although more specifically with regard to a lack of consultation over staffing issues, along with the need for greater access to medical resources, both in terms of time and continuity. Professional conflicts, both within the District Mental Health Service, generally referred to as 'the hospital', and with other agencies, mainly GPs, were mentioned by one third of respondents in the first study, but did not appear as an issue subsequently. Lack of contact with other professional colleagues was mentioned by a small number of team members.

Overall, what the respondents reported as the most satisfying and dissatisfying aspects of their work were broadly similar in the two studies. Direct client work, along with a growing involvement and interest in developmental activities, were seen as the most prominent and positive features, with working as part of a team, one which offered support and encouragement, also seen as a specific source of satisfaction. Most dissatisfactions were focused around the limited availability of both resources and managerial support in the first study, and the proposed general changes in the provision of health and social care in the second study.

Such findings are scarcely surprising; they highlight the positive and negative features of change (Marris, 1986). Whilst organizational changes brought the Cosham team increased opportunities for joint work and a chance to contribute to new developments in service provision, they were invariably accompanied by a level of uncertainty about how and by whom decisions concerning priorities and workload management should be made, in the context of limited resources. Issues were thus implicitly raised about the changing nature of professional practice and the various roles and tasks of each team member.

Team roles and tasks

Concern about the range of skills required to create a more accessible and responsive service was a focus of discussion for the team throughout the period of its development spanned by our study. Whilst welcoming opportunities for professional development, most team members expressed a degree of uncertainty at different times about the changing nature of their roles and tasks. This was evident both from discussions at the regular business meetings and workshops, as reported in Chapter 1, and from the systematic examination of staff attitudes over time presented in the preceding section.

To explore this particular area in more detail, we sought team members' perceptions of their areas of experience, expertise and competence by means of a questionnaire. In addition, each respondent was asked to identify areas of special interest and what they saw as their main training needs. Finally, they were asked to consider how these personal needs and interests related to those of the service as a whole. Once again this exercise was undertaken on two separate occasions: immediately prior to the first stage of the move and again after the whole service had become established in its community base. Although some broad comparisons can be made between the first and second studies, it is important to note once again that there had been a number of individual staff changes in the intervening period.

Professional qualifications

Of the eighteen team members who completed the relevant questionnaire in the first study, fourteen, including ten then based at Vinten House, held a professional nursing qualification in mental health. Three of the staff with nursing qualifications held CPN certificates. The remaining four team members held professional qualifications in occupational therapy, clinical psychology or social work (2). In the follow-up study, after the whole service had moved to Acorn Lodge, seventeen team members completed the questionnaire. Fourteen, nine of them based in the residential unit, held a nursing qualification. Three team members, all based in the community office, held CPN certificates. The three other participating team members were the senior OT and two social workers, who all held professional qualifications. (The clinical psychologist was on maternity leave at the time of the second study.)

In addition to acquiring a professional qualification, each team member had subsequently continued to participate in further education and training, and the wide range of courses reported reflected the diversity of interests across the team. All team members holding a professional nursing qualification had undertaken some additional training in counselling, although this varied in both content and time commitment.

The team members holding other professional qualifications had also participated in a range of post-qualifying training, the content of which reflected similar interests to those of colleagues trained as nurses: developing counselling and psychotherapeutic skills.

Areas of experience and expertise

In response to a question about their perceived strengths in this sense, all team members on both occasions indicated some degree of professional experience and expertise in direct intervention with clients. This was most often referred to in terms of general competence rather than specific skills. The latter were frequently mentioned as areas of possible achievement, through further training in, for example, specific approaches to counselling, groupwork, family therapy, and/or work with people who had been sexually abused. The possession of skills associated with teaching and supervision were also mentioned by most team members.

Approximately half of the respondents on both occasions, seven in the first study and eight in the second, also identified some areas of growing personal expertise. These were largely based on experience, and were focused around developing services and managing a changing organization. These two sub-groups of respondents, not surprisingly, recorded a diversity of interests and a wide range of training needs. Some of these were associated with direct interventions with clients, for example motivational interviewing, behavioural approaches and family therapy; others related to developing and managing services in the community.

Overlapping interests

In response to a question about areas of overlap between their individual professional interests and those of the service as a whole, all team members identified direct work with clients as an area of shared concern. Given the need to develop a flexible, broadly-based, client-orientated service, it was possible for each team member to identify her/his particular contribution within this spectrum of services. Having a degree of flexibility to respond to the changing needs of clients was specifically mentioned by three team members.

Once again, however, the responses could be divided into those which focused more specifically around direct work with clients and those which appeared more broadly based. A group of eleven respondents in the first study, and nine in the second, felt that their interests overlapped with those of the overall service through their contribution to direct work with individual clients. Amongst this group there were some team members who were quite specific about their wish to acquire additional psychotherapeutic skills. This group also identified teaching skills as highly relevant to the development and maintenance of good quality practice throughout the service.

The other group of respondents, seven and eight respectively in the two studies, in addition to noting the appropriateness of developing their therapeutic skills, identified other areas of interest and expertise relevant to the overall needs of the service. Several comments recorded in the first study illustrated this wide range of interests and related training needs. For example:

> *I want to develop management skills and some expertise in behaviour therapy; these relate quite closely to identified needs within the service.*
>
> *Developing continuing care involves direct and indirect client work and relates to acknowledged priorities within the service.*
>
> *They relate very closely ... I want to work with colleagues, managers, users of the service, and other agencies in developing a quality community service.*

These quotations from a number of team members, from several different professional backgrounds, illustrate how each saw the service evolving in a number of ways to meet the diverse needs of a range of people with mental health problems. Similar comments were evident in the second study, along with a growing recognition of changing priorities within the service, as the following statement illustrates:

> *My interests directly relate to the needs of the service, as the needs of the clients with long-term mental health problems/difficulties are, at long last, the focus of our skills - being the relevant area that has been highlighted in the service's overall objectives. It is therefore important to specialize and develop specific skills to be able to meet the needs of this client group and to be able to offer them quality, expertise, experience and knowledge that is their right - so long denied in the past. It is also necessary to be a professional resource for other services: professionals, volunteers, family, and the public; to assist in the development of other more normal resources for these clients, thus enabling further interaction and choice.*

These views were not, however, shared by all respondents, as this comment by another team member suggests:

> *I feel we are being pushed to alter our priorities in some respects ... the move to ensure we are seeing ill people, rather than perhaps counselling at the early stages of distress, to avoid illness.*

Similarities between the two sets of responses - before and after the move to a community base - are readily identifiable, despite the several changes in the service over the intervening period and the increasing emphasis on developing services for continuing care clients. All the respondents on both occasions expressed an interest in, and a felt need to develop, specialist skills associated with direct client interventions. Approximately half also identified a need to develop skills in working with other organizations and networks in the development of services.

Further examination of the two sets of responses revealed some differences with respect to a number of inter-related factors: professional qualifications, work-base, and work experience to date. Of those respondents who wished to focus more specifically on developing practice skills in order to become more effective in their direct work with clients, all spent a substantial proportion of time engaged in assessment work and short-term intervention and all held a nursing qualification; those staff based in the residential unit were highly represented in this group. The second group of respondents, who recorded a more diverse range of interests and associated training needs, were primarily, although not exclusively, those team members who were working with continuing care clients and/or had a co-ordinating aspect to their role. This group included staff from nursing, social work and occupational therapy backgrounds.

Whilst these findings must be treated with caution, they suggest a differential impact on individual team members as the service became more firmly established in the local community. Team members formally identified as working with continuing care clients or having some recognized co-ordinating aspect to their work, having acquired some experience of work in these areas, appeared keen to acquire further expertise in working with others in the development of new services, as well as to extend their skills in direct work with individual clients and their families. For team members primarily based within the residential unit, but increasingly involved in assessment and short-term work with individuals, there appeared to be an equally keen interest in acquiring more specialist skills in such areas. Interestingly, there were very few comments made by any of this group of respondents about either the possession of or the need to develop skills specifically in working with clients in a community-based residential setting.

Summary

This chapter began by noting the far-reaching implications for professional practice of pursuing strategies such as that in Portsmouth to decentralize adult mental health care. We have seen that in many ways staff attitudes as such appear to have changed very little as the Cosham service moved to and began its further development in a community base. The view of the service as being appropriately based on a multidisciplinary area community mental health team, working with and alongside other service providers in their locality - essentially the picture enshrined in the overall strategy of decentralization of mental health services as outlined in the

District Plan - was and remained broadly accepted and shared by the front-line professionals implementing the new approach. However, the staff expressed less clarity and unanimity concerning both decision-making within the team and the types of skills required to develop a community-based service. On these aspects there was evidence of differences of view within the team and of changes over time. Further exploration of staff views on the need to acquire a range of new skills also revealed some differences amongst team members. These latter variations reflected to a considerable extent the different roles and tasks associated with particular practitioners' work within the existing division of labour.

In the concluding discussion which constitutes Chapter 7, the foregoing findings about staff views, which raise central issues concerning professional practice and management in a decentralized setting, will be brought together with our findings on other aspects of the developing service, which have been presented in earlier chapters.

7 Discussion and pointers for the future

Introduction

Whilst the movement towards community care and deinstitutionalization which was embarked upon in the 1950s has generally been sustained, there has been a growing emphasis over the last decade and more, in Britain and elsewhere, on 'providing the best possible service within necessarily limited resources'. Lavender and Holloway (1988, p. 3) summarize the recent past and the current context as follows:

> The movement to establish community care is not new. During the past four decades hospital staff have been discharging people energetically from the large mental hospitals. However, in the latter half of the 1970s and 1980s the movement to provide community-based services has received fresh impetus from the attempt of government and regional health authorities to close these hospitals. This impetus is due to both a genuine desire to improve the quality of the service and an equally genuine desire that the replacement services should be cheaper.

What Lavender and Holloway refer to as 'these mixed motives' in the philosophical and political arguments for 'care in the community', ensure that the development of good quality community mental health services constitutes a major challenge for policy makers, planners and direct service providers alike, particularly with more widespread understanding that this is not necessarily a cheap option and when restricting public expenditure is given high priority in the policies of national governments.

The research reported here set out to examine the organizational and practice issues involved in the process of implementing a policy of 'community care' for people with mental health problems in one particular locality: roughly one third of a large city in Southern England. In presenting our data we have sought to address a rather general question: 'What is the nature and impact of this transition of services from the hospital into the community?' More specifically, and recognizing the transition to be an extended process, we have approached this mainly from the following perspective: 'What can we learn about the impact of this process on those who provide the day-to-day service and those who use it?', acknowledging also that such provision and use involves several groups of people with a variety of interests and concerns.

This book, like the evaluative study on which it is based, has been organized around a series of six formally-stated research aims, set out in full in our Introduction. Each identified aim broadly pointed to one substantial area of investigation, pertinent to the process of implementing a strategy of decentralizing services into local community bases. Chapters 1 - 6 have presented data which in each case focus primarily upon one of the aims and areas of interest. Given the diverse nature of the service studied, and our particular approach to evaluation, there is inevitably and appropriately a degree of overlap between and among the stated aims of the research, the broad areas of investigation arising from them, and the several related, but more specific, service issues involved.

Our six original research aims provide a framework for the first part of this concluding chapter. Each aim is discussed in turn, but now drawing together the material from earlier chapters to offer an overall evaluation of the developing Cosham Mental Health Service over the period of our research and to reflect the main issues and concerns of the service during that time.

The decentralization of the service away from the parent hospital, its diversification, associated with the integration of its community and residential components, and its collaborative activities in association with other local services, are dominant themes throughout the following discussion, in which the views and experiences of those who provide the day-to-day service and those who use it are given a prominent place. A number of issues which reflect the changing nature of professional practice are raised, and the book concludes with more detailed consideration of specific aspects of these themes, highlighting areas which are of current general concern and which need further investigation and action.

Discussion of research aims

Aim 1: To examine how the organization and operation of the Cosham team relates to the overall District strategy for the transition of services into the community.

In 1985, a Unit Manager for Mental Health Services was appointed in Portsmouth, in line with the recommendations of the first Griffiths Report (DHSS, 1983b). A set of guiding principles and some preparatory planning and reorganization towards the decentralization of the service predated this important change, from which the process received fresh impetus.

It was evident from the outset that in attempting 'to operationalize a general philosophy' across the District, similar issues would have to be addressed in each local area. Each multidisciplinary team would be translating the general philosophy into a particular locally-based service, aiming to be widely accessible to its various users and to meet a broad range of needs, including those of people with longer-term mental health problems. The development of a community-based team as the focus for both the organization and the delivery of services would also make consideration of the role of the residential unit within the overall service an important priority.

Our retrospective examination of the early phases of the implementation of the Health Authority's strategic plan, and our more detailed overview of the development of adult mental health services in Cosham during a two-year study period (Chapter 1), showed clearly that a delicate balance between local initiatives and a District-wide framework for community-based services was in fact much in evidence throughout. Thus within an overall strategy of decentralization, both opportunism and innovation were encouraged in bringing about substantial changes in the service as it was moving from hospital to community: still an ongoing process in the Portsmouth Health District. The early variations between the three city teams reflected differences in emphasis in response to local context, rather than fundamentally different patterns of overall organization. Initially, the individuality of the three area teams was encouraged, and within the overall framework local innovations were possible.

Such developments were important not only in effecting change at a local level, but also in contributing towards the achievement of the longer-term goal of overall decentralization. However, some consolidation of these local activities, along with a need to develop a degree of co-ordination across the city, was acknowledged around the time of the commencement of our study with the appointment of a City Manager to replace the three local Area Managers. This trend towards a city-wide service, particularly in the context of developing provision for continuing care clients, was maintained throughout the study period, although various local initiatives within each of the teams also continued to develop.

In its attempts further to improve its accessibility, the Cosham team adopted broadly similar strategies to those of the other teams in the city. It introduced an open referral system and attempted to foster links with other local agencies and organizations, particularly in the early stages of developing better services for people with continuing care needs. However, unlike the team in Southsea, an area where a substantial number of people with longer-term mental health problems had been identified from early on, the Cosham team did not formally identify a sub-group, the Cosham Continuing Care Group, to work in this field until after the first phase of its move to a community base.

A major influence on the early development of the Cosham team as a whole was the particular need to address the question of the relationship between the community and residential aspects of the overall community-based service. Maintaining a division between the two was not really an option for this team, since Vinten House, the residential unit serving the Cosham area, had been set up prior to the establishment of the decentralization strategy, specifically as a way of providing a continuum of care for clients, overcoming the traditional split between residential and community work. What the new Cosham service had to struggle with was the integration of two overlapping but in many ways discrete parts of a total service, which in the early phase of the transition maintained two separate bases within the hospital grounds.

In the interim report on our study (Powell and Lovelock, 1989a) we commented on the pace of change with which service providers were having to cope; this continued to be a prominent feature throughout the remaining period of the research. In part this reflected national policies; in part it resulted from the radical nature of Portsmouth's own strategy. We are inclined to the view that the implementation of the latter was, in a positive sense, to some extent in advance of the former. Be that as it may, the impact of 'permanent revolution' on front-line professionals and managers should not be underestimated.

The introduction of a management structure of the kind advocated for the National Health Service by Griffiths (DHSS, 1983b) and endorsed by the Government, brought additional dimensions of rapid and radical change to those represented by the local decentralization strategy itself. During the latter part of our two-year study, further major nationwide changes appeared on the horizon, particularly through the publication of the White Papers *Working for Patients* (DoH, 1989a) and *Caring for People* (DoH, 1989b), with the latter representing the Government's response to a second report by Sir Roy Griffiths: *Community Care: Agenda for Action* (1988). The speed with which the subsequent NHS and Community Care Bill passed into legislation again serves to underline the pace of change in recent years.

However, there had been an eighteen-month delay - some said 'blight' - between Griffiths' report on community care and the White Paper. This was widely regarded as due to the efforts of the Prime Minister and some of her senior Cabinet colleagues to find an alternative to enhancing the role of local authorities, for Griffiths had recommended that social services departments be given lead responsibility for social as distinct from health care provision, both for people with mental health problems and for other priority groups. Then, some months after the setting of an initial date of April 1991 for full implementation of the NHS and Community Care Act 1990, it was announced that some of the latter's significant sections concerning community care would only come into operation on 1 April 1992, and others not until April 1993. Crucially, this last-mentioned date was set for changes in the funding arrangements regarding residential care for elderly people, the escalating cost of which was widely held to have generated the whole exercise. Further, by the time of finalizing the text of this book, it had been acknowledged by Government that fully developing the new approaches implied by such concepts as case/care management will require a more extended time-scale.

Significant elements of the 1990 Act in respect of service arrangements for people with mental health problems did, however, come into effect on 1 April 1991, so that whilst we were concluding our research and preparing our final report, planning for the implementation of the Act became a major focus of activity for the staff and managers with whom we had been working. District-wide changes in the overall management of Portsmouth's mental health services during the late spring of 1990 reflected the impending national changes, including the requirement that from April 1991 district health authorities and social services departments would have to produce 'formal agreements' in relation to plans for 'an explicit package of services within the scope of the grant' for the 'social care [of] people with a mental illness', and submit them to regional health authorities in order to 'trigger' payment of the new 'Mental Illness Specific Grant' to social services departments. (Department of Health Draft Circular: *Specific Grant for the Development of Social Care Services for People with a Mental Illness*, May 1990). As an interim arrangement, the City Manager in Portsmouth became Acting Unit Manager, prior to taking up the new post of Care Manager (Adult Mental Health Services). At the same time, a Co-ordinators Group was established to manage services across the city. This group, chaired by the Co-ordinator of City Services/Chief Nurse, included representatives from the three city teams and Southsea's continuing care team, a senior nurse psychotherapist, and an administrative officer.

These recent national and local changes further exemplify how continuous change was a feature of the context in which the service being studied was developing during the period of our evaluation. Planning for change and managing change are important themes to which we shall return in our concluding discussion.

Aim 2: To describe and evaluate the overall nature of the Cosham service as a comprehensive community-based facility.

From our descriptive account of the developing Cosham Mental Health Service over time (Chapter 2), it was evident that an increasingly diverse range of activities was being provided within an overall framework. Whilst this does not necessarily indicate that the service is even now a fully comprehensive one, it does suggest that it became increasingly broadly-based and continued to evolve.

The establishment of a community base incorporating a residential unit was unique to this team amongst the three serving the city. This integration was satisfactorily achieved only over an extended period of time. Initial resistance in some quarters was largely replaced by active support (Chapter 1), as demonstrated through the successful introduction of a twenty-four-hour admission policy in June 1990. The new building, which became the work-base of the whole service, came to provide an important focus for many different kinds of activity and facilitated interaction between the numerous members of the multidisciplinary team.

The long-standing and non-traditional community role of those staff based in the residential unit serving Cosham was clearly illustrated by the logging studies reported in Chapter 2, highlighting an important area of overlap between the different aspects of the overall service in this local area. The increasing involvement with non-residents, both at home and at Acorn Lodge, of the staff based in the residential unit, was confirmed in our study of new referrals to the service, reported in Chapter 4.

Another aspect of the increasing diversity of activities taking place within the overall service was the setting up and growing significance of the Cosham Continuing Care Group. The expansion of services available for people with longer-term mental health problems was evident both from our logging studies (Chapter 2) and from our more detailed examination of the emergence of the CCCG (Chapter 3).

To a considerable extent, these areas of development were sustained by the greater involvement of support workers, both within the residential unit and in the day-to-day running of services for continuing care clients. The increasing use of non-professionally qualified staff was evident from our updated account of daily life in the residential unit (Chapter 2), and from our description of day care services for continuing care clients (Chapter 3). This move towards the greater use of support staff has significant implications for professional practice.

Aim 3: To examine the various roles and tasks of the multidisciplinary team as they evolve in the provision of the service.

Changes and developments in service policy and provision are inevitably mirrored in the day-to-day practice of front-line professionals. Whilst direct work with clients continued to be an important focus of activity for all members of the Cosham team, there was evidence, both from the detailed descriptive account of their work (Chapter 2) and from individual accounts of practice (Chapter 3), that many team members were extending their activities to other areas, for example the setting up and running of new service initiatives. The establishment of the CCCG provides the clearest example of how some team members evolved new ways of working, both with individual clients and with other workers in the local community, during the period of our research.

All members of the overall Cosham team saw their direct work with clients as a continuing area of activity, and shared a wish to further develop specialist counselling skills, primarily in one-to-one working, although not exclusively so. Some staff expressed more specific interests in developing skills in working with people who had been sexually abused, or with poorly-motivated clients with longer-term needs (Chapter 6).

Most team members shared a view of the service as being appropriately based on a multidisciplinary team approach and requiring collaboration with other agencies and local networks. However, there was rather less consensus on the types of skills required to meet the challenge of providing a comprehensive community-based service. To some extent this diversity of views reflected the different experiences and interests of team members and individuals' assessments of their particular training needs (Chapter 6).

Some team members viewed the development needs of the overall service and their own professional training needs as significantly interwoven. They were keen to gain further expertise in working with others in the development of new services, and at the same time wanted to extend their skills in direct work with individuals and their families. This overlap in service goals and professional goals was most evident in the views of members of the CCCG, possibly reflecting the work which they had done together in identifying the types of skills required to improve provision for the clients concerned (Chapter 3).

One increasingly significant activity undertaken by most team members, in one form or another, was the supervision of either students engaged in professional training - mainly student nurses - or of the growing number of support workers. This had a day-to-day impact in various ways on individual team members. For example, the role of the duty therapist in the residential unit in providing day-to-day supervision of the support workers was evident from our updated account of the service (Chapter 2). Supervision was also an important task undertaken by the Assistant Clinical Manager in her more formal managerial role within the residential unit.

To a large extent, successfully involving support staff in the maintenance and development of a service, as in Cosham, depends upon the quality of supervision provided by professionally qualified team members. In turn, the latter also need the support which comes from competent and appropriate supervision. Thus the acquisition of skills in giving and indeed receiving staff supervision becomes a particularly important area of professional development in the context of a developing service. This was indicated by the views of several team members quoted in Chapter 6.

Whilst all team members were in broad agreement about the value of multidisciplinary teamwork, both to the users of the service and to themselves, there appeared to be a substantial lack of clarity about decision-making in this context. This was evident from the range of views expressed about the extent to which it was appropriate for all team members to contribute equally to the decision-making process (Chapter 6). This was also the area where there was most evidence of change in the team's views over the period of the study.

The team's difficulty in responding to the growing number of competing demands made on the service, evident from our account of the team's business meetings throughout the study period (Chapter 1), was a further indication of their uncertainty about how and by whom decisions concerning priorities and workload can and should be made. This could already be highlighted as an area of concern in our interim report (Powell and Lovelock, 1989a), and we shall return to it in our concluding discussion.

Aim 4: To explore the relationships and collaborative links established with other locally-based agencies and informal networks in the area.

Our examination of the relationships between the Cosham Mental Health Service and the local area centre of Hampshire Social Services Department (Chapter 3) identified several areas of overlap and collaborative activity between the two agencies. One important initiative was the more systematic involvement of an area centre representative in the Cosham Mental Health Team's weekly allocation meeting. This can be seen as a significant development in the fostering of links between the two services, possibly providing a basis for closer collaboration in future joint service initiatives.

A comparison of data acquired by monitoring referrals to the local area centre (Chapter 3) with that from an analysis of twelve months' referrals to the Cosham Mental Health Team (Chapter 4), raises important issues about provision for people with longer-term mental health problems. Whereas only a small proportion of the referrals to the area centre where a mental health component had been identified either by the referrer or by area staff were recorded as coming from a primary health care team, almost all referrals to the Cosham Mental Health Team were from GPs. There were relatively few self-referrals or referrals by relatives to the Cosham Mental Health Team, and amongst the whole group of referrals to the latter, practical difficulties were given prominence only in a small number of instances. Conversely, referrals to the area centre included a number of people who were identified by social workers as having a mental health component to their difficulties, and who had referred themselves or had been referred by relatives for advice and/or for help with various practical problems such as accommodation and finance. Given the nature of their difficulties, this group may have represented or included a proportion of the people with continuing mental health care needs in the area who may not have been in direct contact with or known to the Cosham Mental Health Service. Moreover, our interview material, particularly that from discussions with GPs (Chapter 5), suggested that people with longer-term mental health problems tended to have little contact with their family doctors.

An important joint initiative to develop a more accessible form of service for people with longer-term mental health problems was the setting up of an informal drop-in facility: the Sevenoaks Club. Given the genuinely joint nature of developments such as this, it matters little whether potential members first come to the attention of the social services area centre or the mental health service. In outlining the setting up and early operation of this club (Chapter 3), we drew attention to a number of features which possibly contributed to its early success as a collaborative venture between the statutory agencies and a voluntary organization. It may be seen as one very good example of a local innovation which has embodied collaboration and partnership between the statutory and independent sectors. As such it provides an example at 'street level' of what Griffiths (1988) envisaged as the future pattern of community care.

Although creating closer links with GPs was on the agenda for the Cosham team throughout, there was little substantial development on this front during our study period (Chapter 1). One successful example of regular contact between the Cosham team and a particular group practice did, however, become well-established, although our interviews with GPs, reported in Chapter 5, suggested that its transferability might be limited. Whilst the GPs we interviewed generally confirmed the need for closer working relationships between primary health care teams and specialist mental health services, they also indicated the difficulties which remain to be overcome.

One initiative, not discussed in detail in the main body of this text since it was only in its early stages at the time our final report on the study (Powell and Lovelock, 1991) was being prepared, was the establishment of a duty officer team, following a further review of the arrangements for duty cover. An important facet of this development was its emphasis on achieving closer working links with GPs, both on an individual basis in the context of responding to specific referrals and in a more general way with group practices as such. Within the duty officer team, the importance of a regular contribution from the medical staff was emphasized. The team's recognition of the need actively to involve one of its medical members at this initial stage of a client's contact with the service reflected some of the concerns expressed by GPs, including to the researchers in interview (Chapter 5). This also represents one way in which psychiatrists can actively contribute to a team initiative.

Aim 5: To identify and describe the various categories of service user.

The vast majority of the people newly referred to the service over the twelve-month period analyzed in detail (Chapter 4) were referred by their GPs. Anxiety and/or depression figured predominantly as identified forms of distress for which specialist help was sought on these clients' behalf. Whilst the number of referrals each month remained relatively stable, twice as many women as men were referred and two-thirds of the people concerned were not previously known to the service.

In the majority of cases, the initial response to a referral was a team discussion, followed by one team member - sometimes two jointly - seeking direct contact with the client for further assessment and discussion of possible ways of helping. Taking this action on behalf of the service was increasingly shared among all members of the team. Clinical decisions concerning the appropriateness of a therapeutic intervention for individual service users thus to some extent became acknowledged as a team responsibility (Chapter 4).

Regular weekly referral/assessment meetings provided a forum for the deliberations of the team, although discussion there tended to focus substantially more on the allocation of cases than on their continued oversight (Chapter 1). The latter took place more in the context of one-to-one staff supervision, and was generally more concerned with ensuring good practice than with providing a means of accountability.

In approximately 10 per cent of referrals an urgent response to a perceived crisis was sought by a GP. In these situations the form of help required was generally a medical assessment and access to specialist medical help or the use of residential care. Whilst there were examples of the duty officer system being used in this context, access to the consultant psychiatrist via a formal request for a domiciliary visit was the preferred mechanism and the more commonly employed route to help.

Although GPs continued to play an important role as gatekeepers in these and other referral situations, self-referral to the service was encouraged, not least (Chapter 3) in the context of service initiatives for continuing care clients, where ways of being both more accessible and more acceptable to these users were explored. The Sevenoaks Club, specifically set up as an informal drop-in facility, is one important example of this, and has already been referred to in this chapter in discussing collaborative ventures. It attempted to encourage people with longer-term mental health problems to make contact and to keep in touch: both people not previously known to the service or whose contact has lapsed, and those currently in contact with the service. Because of its informal nature, only very crude quantitative indicators of the club's use by its membership were available. However, club members' views about the service provide an important qualitative indication of its success (Powell, 1991).

Aim 6: To assess, from the various 'consumer' perspectives, the overall impact of the service on its direct users, their relatives, and relevant professional and other groups and services.

The foregoing discussion of aim 5 concentrated on direct service users. However, we have been at pains throughout to use the term 'service users' in an inclusive way, and to refer both to caring relatives or friends and to professionals outside the Cosham Mental Health Service as in different senses users of the services provided by the specialist staff team. Exploring these various users' views and experiences concerning the quality and impact of the service formed an important part of our overall evaluation of it, enabling the identification of the extent to which its underlying principles, outlined in Chapter 1, were evident in its day-to-day operation.

Our interviews indicated that, for all groups of users, both accessibility and acceptability were key dimensions of their overall assessment of the service. Where a choice of venues for direct contact had been offered, this had been greatly appreciated. Contact in the home was also highly valued, alongside the availability of a range of facilities and services in the locality.

For the vast majority of newly-referred users and their GPs, the service, whilst relatively narrowly perceived as providing counselling help, was regarded as satisfactory and meeting a growing demand for such forms of intervention (Chapter 5). The increasing demand from their patients for help with emotional distress, and a desire to seek alternatives to medication, encouraged most GPs to use the more locally accessible and acceptable service as a counselling facility rather than as a specialist psychiatric service. Whilst their GP was usually seen as having initiated the possibility of contact with the Cosham team, most of the people referred felt that there had been a process of negotiation, before a formal request by the GP was made to the service (Chapter 5).

Users of the Sevenoaks Club and of the contact clubs were relatively well-informed about the range of facilities contributing to the overall service (Chapter 3). They had often had both contact with one or more of the clubs and some involvement with a particular team member. They welcomed access to both forms of help, valuing each as an important contribution to their continued well-being.

Interestingly, these users raised issues concerning the changing role of their key workers and the increasing prominence of volunteers and non-professional staff in the day-to-day running of the social clubs. They welcomed these developments, provided that access to professional support was available when needed. These observations by the users of the continuing care services confirmed those made by some staff belonging to the Cosham Continuing Care Group on their changing patterns of practice (Chapter 3), which were highlighted in our account of the operation of the overall service (Chapter 2).

One area of concern raised by some GPs, and confirmed by the views of some direct users and their relatives (Chapters 3 and 5), was the difficulty sometimes experienced in engaging and sustaining contact with potential users, particularly those poorly motivated to seek help. This is relevant to any consideration of the training needs of team members, and was also specifically mentioned by some members of the Cosham team as a growing area of interest (Chapter 6).

These findings, along with those indicating patterns of service use (Chapter 4), raise issues about the appropriate role of the Cosham team and the relative balance between providing a much-needed counselling service for users referred by GPs, a specialist service able to respond to immediate requests for help with acute 'psychiatric emergencies', and the development of services for people with longer-term mental health problems. Maintaining a balance between these different aspects of the overall service, through negotiating boundaries with other agencies and setting priorities within the service, became an increasingly pressing concern as the Cosham Mental Health Service developed in the community. This was identified as an issue in our interim report (Powell and Lovelock, 1989a) and the additional findings from the later stages of the study further highlighted the important substantive questions involved, along with how and by whom decisions should be made on these matters.

A related question, and one about which some GPs expressed concern, was that of accountability. The view of a small number of GPs that the consultant psychiatrist should hold a position of team leader, was generally expressed with reference to seeking an immediate response to a perceived crisis, where access to medical resources or residential care was being sought. The revised duty officer team arrangements, referred to above as having been adopted after the completion of our study, may prove valuable here, not least in clearly identifying a role for medical staff in these situations.

Some direct users perceived the overall service as being co-ordinated by the doctor, although this largely reflected the experiences of particular individuals. Many users had little clear idea of who might be in charge, or perhaps more importantly to whom a complaint might be made. Whilst this issue was not felt very significant by most users, some assumed that if such a need arose they would seek the advice of their GP. The uncertainty expressed by a small number of GPs regarding overall responsibility within the team for clinical matters, indicates that this whole area is potentially a difficult one. It is, however, an important aspect of the process of involving users in the development of local services.

Our interviews (Chapters 3 and 5) indicated clearly that having some account taken of their own views and experiencing an active involvement in the 'helping process' contributed substantially to direct users' satisfaction with the service. For those participating in counselling, this was expressed in terms of being 'enabled' or 'empowered'. For users of the continuing care services, a sense of involvement came rather from their experience of being able to choose what activities they wished to participate in, or sometimes whether they had to participate at all; some also mentioned their positive experiences of being able to join in and to take some responsibility for the day-to-day planning of activities.

User involvement in the overall management and planning of services is still very much in its infancy. In the context of the Cosham Mental Health Service it was confined during our study period to a few aspects of the service, for example the Sevenoaks Club Management Committee, but was clearly on the agenda for the future.

Summary

So far in this concluding chapter, we have drawn together the research findings presented in earlier chapters and thereby systematically addressed each of our stated research aims and the service issues to which they relate. Not only is there a considerable degree of interlinking between these aims and issues; the different sorts and sources of data upon which we have drawn are also mutually supportive. We are now, therefore, in a position to offer an overall assessment of the achievements of the Cosham Mental Health Service during the phase in its development which we studied.

A broad strategy, consisting of some general service principles and a statement of the essential organizational structure for a District-wide service which would be firmly based in the local community which it serves rather than on a large and segregated hospital site, provided a flexible framework for development. Within this, multidisciplinary teams serving the three areas of Portsmouth were able to identify and respond to needs in ways reflecting their varying local contexts, developing both their direct work with clients and their involvement in service initiatives. It became necessary to consolidate and co-ordinate local initiatives by increasing the city-wide nature of the service, particularly with regard to developing provision for continuing care clients.

The Cosham service was broadly-based from early on and became increasingly diverse and comprehensive. This was recognized by both staff and users. The Cosham team's main preoccupation during the early phase of its transition was with bringing together its community and residential roles and staff groups. Despite particular and perhaps unique difficulties in this respect, by the end of the period of our study this integration had been achieved to a very large degree. This essentially followed the relocation of the service as a whole in one building away from the hospital site. The overall Cosham team had begun to give detailed attention to developing services for continuing care clients in advance of this, but not to any great extent during the first year of our research. The increasing diversification of the service was reflected throughout the study period in the changing roles and tasks evident amongst the multidisciplinary team. Non-professionally qualified staff came to play an increasingly important role in several aspects of the overall service.

The development of a drop-in facility for people with longer-term mental health problems was a very significant joint initiative, involving the community mental health team, staff from the local social services area centre, and colleagues from voluntary agencies. There was also increasing collaboration with area-based social work staff in other ways; for example, a representative of the area team attended the mental health team's weekly referral/allocation meetings from early on. However, at the end of our study there appeared to be scope for further work to ensure the early identification of people with mental health problems and their referral to the most appropriate agency, and for cross-referral, particularly in respect of people with longer-term mental health needs, who commonly encounter a number of additional practical problems.

The vast majority of new referrals to the Cosham Mental Health Service over the two-year period of our study continued to come from GPs. The most common recorded reason for referral throughout a period of one year analyzed in detail was anxiety and/or depression, and the monthly referral rate was fairly constant. Response to these referrals was increasingly a task spread amongst the whole team, including residential staff, after a team discussion. In a small proportion of cases a more urgent response was made, by a medical team member in almost half of the instances, often in answer to a specific formal request for a psychiatric assessment.

For direct users, relatives, and GPs, accessibility and acceptability were key features of largely positive evaluations of the new-style service. They also shared a tendency to see the service essentially as providing much-valued counselling as an alternative to medication in response to emotional distress. The relationships and boundaries between the primary health care team and the specialist mental health service were recognized as needing further attention. Some preliminary efforts had been made in terms of links with specific practices.

We observed the beginnings of user involvement in the service. Clients in our interview sample of new referrals felt that their approach to the service had been the outcome of a process of negotiation with their GP. They greatly appreciated the availability of a range of local facilities and the choice of venue for the receipt of help which the Cosham staff offered them, including in particular the possibility of meeting in clients' own homes. They felt 'enabled' by support and counselling. Continuing care clients felt involved in the day-to-day running of the drop-in centre and contact clubs and had begun to play a role in their management.

An extension and diversification of team members' activities led to them feeling a need to acquire additional skills, both in direct work with clients and in collaborating with colleagues, including those in other agencies, to develop services. Some users, GPs, and members of the Cosham team identified a need for special attention to making and sustaining contact with poorly-motivated clients.

Staff experienced a lack of clarity with regard to decision-making, particularly in the areas of priority-setting and workload management. In addition, some GPs and a small number of direct users raised questions about clinical accountability and professional leadership. Staff comments implied a need for attention to professional supervision.

Overall, it may be said that the radical agenda for change set for the Cosham team was substantially addressed during the period in which we studied the development process; major and largely positive developments took place over a relatively short timescale. It is of no little significance that the process of decentralization in Portsmouth has been taking place in a period characterized by major change on a wider scale. In particular, the impact of implementing a Griffiths-style 'general management approach' throughout the NHS was evident within the Cosham Mental Health Service. At the end of our research, further cultural and organizational change was being prepared for in response to the White Papers *Working For Patients* (DoH, 1989a) and *Caring For People* (DoH, 1989b), embodied together in the NHS and Community Care Act 1990, with quite specific intentions regarding mental health services. National changes in primary health care, including new GP contracts, together with a phased restructuring of Hampshire Social Services Department (see p. 199) in response to 'the Griffiths (community care) agenda', all promised to prove significant to the team's ongoing activities and future development.

A number of important issues needing further attention can be identified by reflecting on Portsmouth's developmental initiative. These constitute an agenda for additional work in the future, not only in Portsmouth and Hampshire but elsewhere.

Outstanding issues

Taken together, our findings concerning developments in Portsmouth are consistent with those of other recent research in this field. For example, Lavender and Holloway (1988, pp. 288-9) identify seeking out need rather than waiting for a crisis, offering a broad therapeutic approach - one which is less purely medically-based than in the past - to the problems of clients and their families, and having:

> a range of skilled and well trained staff working in a co-ordinated way that enables them to support each other and provide the user with a high quality service,

as the key features of 'good quality community-orientated services'.

Broadly speaking, the Cosham Mental Health Service as we observed it develop can be said to meet Lavender and Holloway's criteria. We would add that the Portsmouth experience also demonstrates the value of an appropriate overall strategy and organizational structure for district-wide services, providing a broad framework within which local innovation is encouraged, as advocated by Jones (1988, pp. 159-60). This has facilitated the development of diversified and responsive services, not only in the area on which our case study focused, but in other parts of the city.

The areas which our research suggests need further attention by policy makers, service managers and staff also confirm the work of others. For example, Lavender and Holloway (op. cit.) point to setting clear priorities, meeting the training needs generated by changing staff roles and skill requirements, adequate and sensitive supervision, and relationships with GPs and the primary health care team, as the major issues outstanding in the development of good quality community mental health services.

In an attempt to assist such development, we conclude this book with further discussion of these and associated issues in the light of our case study in Portsmouth, under the headings of 'organizational change', 'locally-based services', 'developing professional practice', and 'managing priorities and workload'.

Organizational change

The broad national context Both an adequate level of funding and a clear acknowledgement of where specific lead responsibilities rest are crucial to the development of high quality mental health services. These are areas where national governments have a major responsibility. The extent to which the NHS and Community Care Act 1990 has satisfactorily addressed these issues continues to be debated, sometimes acrimoniously, although implementation has now become the main focus of attention for managers and practitioners. Resource issues and the vexed question of the workability of the distinction and boundaries between health and social care are but two areas where disputes are unlikely to be resolved in the near future to the satisfaction of all concerned. We do not wish to enter directly into these debates here; the passage of the legislation in a sense resolved some questions for the time being, whilst the unfolding of events in practice is the only possible source of answers to others.

Since the White Paper *Caring For People* (DoH, 1989b) appeared late in our research period, and the NHS and Community Care Act 1990 was passed whilst our final report (Powell and Lovelock, 1991) was in preparation, their specific content could not directly influence the study itself. However, a number of the key points emerging from this research might usefully inform the implementation of the Act.

Care in the community We referred earlier in this chapter to the arrangements for accessing the new 'Mental Illness Specific Grant', aimed at generating jointly planned and locally-relevant social care services. It is significant that this is one aspect of the community care legislation which has been operative from April 1991, coupled with another major change, namely the 'Care Programme Approach' (DoH, 1990) required of health authorities in discharging people from hospital. These developments reflect a recognition of the problems which have been experienced in seeking to run down the large old mental hospitals whilst at the same time developing appropriate services in the local community. Many commentators would of course say that the resources required to resolve these difficulties have not been guaranteed, pointing to the numbers of homeless people on the streets of our major cities as evidence.

The Care Programme Approach is actually enshrined in legislation only for people discharged from hospital following mental illness. In general terms it appears to relate closely to the concept of case management, which was officially advocated in *Caring For People* (DoH, 1989b) for the provision of social care services for elderly and physically and mentally disabled people as a whole. However, the relevant guidance documents on the implementation of the new overall community care arrangements (DoH/Scottish Office, 1991), which closely link assessment and care management, indicate differences between the latter and the Care Programme Approach, at least on the Government's favoured model of care management - its now preferred terminology. The following clarification is contained in the *Managers' Guide* (p. 93):

> The major difference between the Care Programme Approach and care management is that, under the former, the key worker may have some responsibility for service delivery whereas this would not normally apply to care management.

How extensively case/care management develops in the context of providing care in the community for people with mental health problems, and what the nature of health, social services and voluntary sector partnership in this area will be, remain to be seen. The provision of social care services, to be arranged by social services departments but not necessarily directly or exclusively provided by the statutory sector, will develop in the shifting context in which all local authority activity currently finds itself. Local assessment systems are to be tested out during 1992/3 and implemented from 1 April 1993 along with the changed financial arrangements for residential care, but it has now been officially acknowledged that a fully-developed care management approach will take some further years to evolve: proposals only are required in 1993/4 community care plans (DoH/Scottish Office, 1991, *Summary*, p. 28). Changes in primary health care, flowing from an earlier White Paper (DHSS, 1987) and including an emphasis on preventive work and health promotion, as well as the major changes in the organization of the health service as a whole (and, as we write, also in a growing number of social services departments) around the purchaser/provider split, are also part of the general context in which further development of community mental health services must proceed.

Further discussion of these issues is beyond the scope of this book. However, in a context of continuing change, there are grounds for concern that preoccupation with overall organizational issues on the part of policy makers and senior managers could lead to the dissipation of the progress made in local contexts such as Cosham towards genuine multidisciplinary working at 'street level'. Not least under threat in this way is the crucial process of referral, assessment, and the flexible provision of individualized services.

Managing change We have suggested that an environment marked by constant and significant change has been the milieu in which Portsmouth's locally-based mental health services have been developing. Planning for change inevitably involves uncertainty. This makes it particularly important both that the links between policy and practice are given close attention and that implementation is conceived and actively pursued as a process necessarily involving an interplay between overall policy and 'street-level' practice. Learning from local innovations and using the lessons from them to promote changes in mainstream practice is of central importance to such a conception of planning for and managing change. Griffiths (1988, p. *iv*, para. 11) highlighted this, and it is widely recognized as a way of encouraging the development of high quality local services (Kingsley and Towell, 1988).

Particularly in a context of rapid and extensive change, it is important that all those involved in providing the new-style services are enabled to take time for constructive reflection on where they as individuals and groups of professionals are going. The basis for this is regular and systematic review of changes occurring over time (Marris, 1986). We believe that our own work alongside the Cosham service during a crucial period in its development has helped to promote this approach (Powell and Lovelock, 1989b, 1992). The front-line service providers involved have acknowledged this; so too have their managers. In our view it is important that opportunities for staff to 'make sense' of their experience in order to learn from it are actively facilitated and sustained in the longer term.

Locally-based services

Models for development The broadly successful decentralization and diversification of the Cosham Mental Health Service has involved both the coming together of the community and residential aspects of the service and the staff groups involved, and the development of collaborative activity and joint working with other local agencies. The setting up of an informal drop-in centre, the Sevenoaks Club, has been highlighted as one particularly successful example of a local joint project (see also Powell, 1991). This initiative, along with others referred to in our detailed discussion of collaborative links (Chapter 3), provides a solid local model for the forms of development envisaged by Griffiths (1988) and endorsed in the NHS and Community Care Act 1990.

The extension of this sort of approach to care in the community represents a significant and substantial task for the future. It is important that local initiatives such as the Sevenoaks Club are publicized further afield as a means of contributing to a wider improvement in the quality of community-based services for people with longer-term mental health problems. Both the information service provided by Good Practices in Mental Health, and the Kings Fund Institute (e.g. Kings Fund Institute, 1987) have offered accounts of such innovative service developments across the UK.

User involvement The perceptions and experiences of a variety of users of the Cosham Mental Health Service have been given some prominence in this book, as an important part of the overall evaluation undertaken. Commissioning such research is one way in which service providers can pay proper attention to service quality and to the interests of consumers, as they are explicitly required to do by the NHS and Community Care Act 1990. Positive aspects of the service can be identified, alongside areas needing further thought and improvement. For example, in our study, users' uncertainties around the issue of accountability highlighted the need to give careful consideration to the setting up of a well-publicized formal complaints procedure, as envisaged in recent legislation.

An important dimension in the setting up of the Sevenoaks Club was the attempt to take account of users' views, both in the day-to-day running of the club and in its overall management. Whilst still in the exploratory stage, such moves towards involving users in the development of services are vital and require sustained effort if 'consumerism' is to be taken seriously. Careful attention has to be given to the variety of ways in which users' views may usefully inform service development, and the likely implications of this for professional practice (Hugman, 1991).

Beresford and Croft (1990b) are among a number of writers who have drawn attention to the variety of quite different philosophies and models which can be used to underpin attempts at 'user involvement' or 'empowerment'. The Open Services Project (Beresford and Croft, 1990a) has explored the variety of ways in which statutory and voluntary agencies are beginning to involve users in the provision of services. Also of interest here is a survey of the views of people with mental health problems about their needs and the services available, carried out in the context of the Birmingham Community Care Special Action Project (Ritchie et al., 1988).

This survey was more broadly-based than was possible in the context of our own study. Good Practices in Mental Health has published a collection of papers describing several substantial examples of user empowerment in mental health services (Barker and Peck, 1987), whilst the Centre for Health Economics at the University of York and the Kings Fund Centre for Health Services Development are also active in this field, particularly in relation to quality assurance.

Links and boundaries with GP services Developments in the setting up of a duty officer team, which took place after our research was complete but whilst we were still in contact with the Cosham Mental Health Service, represented an attempt to address the need for closer working relationships between the latter and local GPs, particularly in responding to urgent requests for specialist help. The role of the general practitioner and the wider primary health care team in the care of people with longer-term mental health problems has not been an area much explored (Jones et al., 1983). The identification of one or more members of a specialist mental health team to act as 'link person(s)' to GP practices might assist in the further clarification of the mutual roles of the former and the latter. Any team members with a particular interest in working at the interface between the two services, and possessing 'reticulist' skills, could make a significant contribution (McKeganey and Hunter, 1986). Furthermore, in the changing context of primary health care, and in the light of the new GP contracts, preventive work and health promotion are very much on the agenda. This has received further impetus from the recent Green Paper *The Health of the Nation* (DoH, 1991b).

Whilst access to counselling facilities was commented upon favourably both by GPs and by the direct beneficiaries of the specialist service which we studied, the predominance of this aspect of the Cosham team's actual or potential contribution in the perceptions of both referrers and clients raises major issues in terms of the comprehensiveness and accessibility of the service to the full range of potential users.

Deciding at whom a specialist service is aimed and thereby identifying priority groups, and keeping this under review, are necessary disciplines if the needs of those with the most severe problems are to be met (Richman and Barry, 1985). An essential part of this process involves establishing appropriate and agreed boundaries between the service and its major partners, in particular GPs and the relevant social services department(s) (Fisher et al., 1984). We shall return to these issues from a different perspective in the next section.

The social services department A number of studies (Huxley et al., 1987; Isaac et al., 1986) have identified considerable psychiatric morbidity among cases seen by social workers in area teams. In this context, establishing closer links with such local professional colleagues can be seen as an area of substantial achievement on the part of the Cosham team during the study period. It is important that such collaborative activities are sustained and promoted in and by both agencies in the context of future developments.

The first phase of an overall restructuring of Hampshire Social Services Department took effect in April 1990, with overarching aims very similar to those lying behind Portsmouth's decentralization of mental health services: namely the provision of a comprehensive and integrated service, more accessible and responsive to users' needs. The proposed new structure was initially outlined as being consistent with the recommendations of the (second) Griffiths Report (1988) and was subsequently promoted as being in tune with the spirit and requirements of the NHS and Community Care Act 1990. Similar changes in organizational structure, with decentralization of service and (often to a lesser degree) financial management, are taking place in social services departments across the UK.

Towell (1985) rightly suggests that social services departments have a major role to play in leading the development of community-based services; there must be social services input at all levels, including in the context of regional policy and planning. However, in our discussion under the heading 'organizational change', we referred to the danger that a primary focus on major structural changes, which often tends to preoccupy senior managers and politicians in this context, could lead to a failure adequately to acknowledge the progress already made at 'street level' and a failure to address the issues of professional practice which require attention in the concrete areas of collaborative working to which the overall strategic changes are ultimately directed. In a similar way it is possible that the attempts in recent White Papers and legislation clearly to identify lead agencies and to distinguish their and other bodies' responsibilities, and to replace exhortations to joint planning with the requirement for specific 'planning agreements', could have a negative effect on further front-line service development.

Opportunities for service development at local level have been facilitated by the Approved Social Worker provisions of the Mental Health Act 1983 and the requirement that a sufficient number of social work staff must be properly trained and accredited to work with people with mental health problems. A recently-published SSI report on ASWs (DoH, 1991a) emphasizes that they have a broad and influential role to play in the development of services, in addition to their vital responsibilities in relation to requests for compulsory admission to hospital.

To sustain joint work such as that undertaken by health and social services agencies in the local situation which we studied, whilst structural changes such as those within Hampshire Social Services Department unfold, it is important that front-line staff committed to working with people with mental health problems are encouraged and enabled to maintain their collaborative activities with other agencies and local networks. This applies both to social workers based in health settings and to their colleagues in area teams. It is particularly important that the developmental work of the growing number of specialist mental health social workers should continue alongside their role as an accessible specialist resource for departmental and other colleagues, and for clients.

Developing professional practice

Identifying skills In the course of implementing a locally-based approach, the Cosham Mental Health Team acquired considerable experience of direct work with clients in a multidisciplinary and community setting and of developing local resources in collaboration with others. It is important that such staff are encouraged to articulate the nature of their changing professional practice, so that a core of practice skills necessary for the development of community-based services may be identified. In the particular setting studied, this process was stimulated to some extent through the activities of review and evaluation undertaken by the Cosham Continuing Care Group. Such reflection could usefully be extended to other areas of innovatory practice.

The articulation of what constitutes 'good practice' is an important step in identifying staff development and training needs and is ultimately a contribution to the establishment of high quality locally-based services. Without this, as Lavender and Holloway (1988, p. 299) point out:

> ... there is no reason to believe that the quality of care outside the traditional institution will be any better than within it.

The Cosham Mental Health Service has provided a pointer for services elsewhere engaged in similar developments.

Moreover, understanding of this sort gained in the mental health field is broadly applicable to other client groups. It should therefore be of considerable interest to all agencies in the social care field as they develop more responsive community-based services. Not least, social services departments should find it relevant as they explore the 'enabling' role which recent legislation foresees for them.

Multidisciplinary teamwork There are several long-standing issues relating to the organization and operation of multidisciplinary teams (Øvretveit, 1986; Øvretveit, Temple and Coleman, 1988; Soni et al., 1989; Iles and Auluck, 1990). Not the least important of these focus around the distinctions and inter-relationships between questions of professional/clinical judgement and managerial authority and accountability, which of course have wider relevance within human services agencies. Particular difficulties on this score arise in multidisciplinary teams, where commonly some of the professions represented have vertical and others horizontal forms of organization. Thus a consultant will have a considerable degree of autonomy - in the immediate context of this discussion we are not concerned as such with the issues around general management within the health service - whilst other team members will be responsible in line management terms to superiors outside the team. The Cosham Mental Health Team is by no means unique in having as an additional factor here that its social workers alone were employed by a different agency from the other members of the team, all of whom, despite their varying professional disciplines, were (and are) employed by the health service. The need for professional supervision and support, and the question of leadership within the team, must be considered as part of this complex of issues.

These well-known themes were evident in earlier evaluated developments within Portsmouth's mental health services (Evans et al., 1986; Powell and Lovelock, 1987a). A good example from the present study of a key issue around which difficulties can and did arise, despite substantial progress being made, is the changing role of the psychiatrist in the context of the multidisciplinary team. Aspects of this have been touched upon at several points in this book, for example concerning the referral process and the move of the residential unit away from the hospital. In setting up its new duty team, after the completion of our study, the Cosham service acknowledged the importance of a regular medical input into the group. However, this contribution was generally understood as primarily one of clinical expertise rather than of 'sapiential leadership' (Soni et al., 1989). As we have seen, how and by whom decisions should be made, both on a day-to-day basis and concerning the overall development of the local service, was an area of uncertainty throughout the study period, and remained an issue demanding careful consideration at all levels of the organization.

Roles and responsibilities One set of issues basic to team organization concerns where responsibility for assessment and treatment decisions are located and how decisions are made and reviewed about treatment programmes (Øvretveit, Temple and Coleman, 1988). Each member of the Cosham team enjoyed a relatively high degree of professional autonomy. A lack of clarity surrounding the issues of accountability and leadership, both within the multidisciplinary team and amongst those professionals and clients in contact with it, contributed to this. The value of involving other team members in joint consultations and shared work was, however, widely accepted and practised. Whilst considerable progress was made in defining individual team members' responsibilities and establishing procedures for the referral and allocation of cases, further work concerning the different but overlapping professional roles appeared important and necessary (NHSHAS/SSI, 1989, pp. 24-5. More generally, see Mittler, 1987; Patmore and Weaver, 1989). In his 1986 paper, Øvretveit provides a useful framework for clarifying certain aspects of team organization, identifying areas related to distinctive professional skills, areas of both overlapping and common professional competence and responsibilities, and specific but non-professional skills.

During our study period, members of the Cosham team were increasingly recognizing supervision of their own work and the work of others, particularly colleagues without professional training, as an important activity. We noted earlier in this chapter that although in the majority of cases initial responses to new referrals followed team discussion, ongoing review tended to be undertaken in the context of individual professional supervision aimed at ensuring good practice, rather than on a team basis and as a mechanism of accountability. Some of the GPs interviewed touched on this area when discussing the issue of team accountability and decision-making.

Although based on social services departments, Clare's observations (1988) regarding the nature of effective supervision, and its crucial role in both the monitoring of client service and the maintenance of practitioners engaged in stressful forms of practice, are relevant here. Future work on the operational policies of teams such as that in Cosham should give careful consideration to relationships and mechanisms of accountability in team members' direct work with clients, as well as to general professional supervision.

Managing priorities and workload

A second key set of organizational issues identified by Øvretveit and his colleagues (1988) concern responsibility for limiting or extending individual and team workloads, and for the setting and changing of service boundaries and priorities. These are questions of overall policy and managerial accountability and authority, rather than being matters of professional or clinical judgement. In the context of services such as those provided by the Cosham Mental Health Team, the main areas to be balanced are specialist psychiatric help, counselling in the broad sense, support for continuing care clients, and general educative and preventive work. To varying degrees, more than direct work with clients is involved in each of these areas.

It is particularly important that in the planning of development initiatives some consideration is given to their impact on other aspects of the service concerned, and that such planning is seen as an ongoing reflective and participative process. During our study period a number of specific service development initiatives took place, each of which had a significant and often largely unforeseen impact on other aspects of the service. In particular, maintaining a balance between the demands - predominantly from GPs - for a counselling service, and those of ongoing work with continuing care clients, gradually and inevitably forced questions upon the team about setting priorities and managing workload.

Determining the priorities of the service and keeping them under review, with consequent limiting or extending of both individual and team workloads, can be seen as a matter both for the team itself and for senior managers (Øvretveit, Temple and Coleman, 1988). These issues were raised as pressing concerns in our interim report (Powell and Lovelock, 1989a), and remained in need of urgent attention at the end of the study period. They are central to the development of effective teamwork and thus of a good quality local service.

Responsibility for setting initial boundaries and objectives, and for clearly articulating them for staff, rests with higher management (Patmore and Weaver, 1991). Meanwhile, the staff team itself has responsibility for defining its own arrangements for managing its agreed workload. The Cosham experience provides some useful pointers for the future.

Portsmouth's City Co-ordinators Group, established as our research drew to a close, may prove to be a useful forum in the context of setting overall service priorities. Having team forums where ideas can be presented and discussed would be one way of encouraging the process by which patch teams work out their own more specific policies and procedures, reflecting local conditions. The use of small working groups within an overall area team to develop particular aspects of policy and practice is another way forward. Such an approach was found of value in Cosham in working towards the establishment of the new duty officer system.

The roles and tasks of a team co-ordinator, particularly in relation to the management of the team's agreed workload, need clear identification and agreement. The Cosham Co-ordinator, as a member of the City Co-ordinator's Group and a key participant in local team meetings and working groups, evolved an important negotiating and mediating function.

Final comments

In outlining a blueprint for 'a good community mental health service', Jones (1988, pp. 159-60) argues the need for a structure which would locate appropriate elements of responsibility firmly at national, local, and individual client levels. Its main characteristics would be:

> diversity, informality, outreach and critical feedback. It combines American know-how, British pragmatism, Italian warmth and something of the pioneering spirit of China in a new model of care.

The decentralizing mental health service which was the focus of the evaluative study reported in this book may be said substantially to exemplify the local and client level dimensions of what is being reached for in Jones' formulation. Although subject to the constraints imposed by limited resources, there was growing diversity within the overall service.

Some aspects of the service showed a highly-developed level of informality; others had made less progress on this front. Outreach activities, embodying collaboration with other agencies and networks, were a growing feature of the service throughout the period of the research. Last, but by no means least, the service's awareness of the importance of critical feedback and of finding ways in which the experience of service development can be used as learning for subsequent initiatives was evidenced by its participation in this study.

As Kingsley and Towell (1988, p. 53) observe, in outlining a model of service development which has considerable affinity with Portsmouth and South-East Hampshire Health Authority's approach to decentralizing its adult mental health services:

> The challenge of planning for new patterns of service is to go beyond existing and known forms of provision. This will require a robust framework for dealing with and adapting to changing circumstances, while always maintaining a clear end in view.

In carrying out evaluative research alongside this process we adopted a similar approach, in order to provide critical but constructive feedback as a contribution to the ongoing process of service development. Thus our account of an attempt in one part of Southern England to implement 'care in the community' for people with mental health problems offers a positive example of what can be achieved and indicates what remains to be done.

References

Audit Commission (1986), *Making a Reality of Community Care*, HMSO, London.
Barker, I. and Peck, E. (eds) (1987), *Power in Strange Places: User Empowerment in Mental Health Services*, Good Practices in Mental Health, London.
Beresford, P. and Croft, S. (1986), *Whose Welfare: Private Care or Public Services?*, Lewis Cohen Urban Studies Centre, Brighton.
Beresford, P. and Croft, S. (1990a), *From Paternalism to Participation: Involving People in Social Services*, Open Services Project/Joseph Rowntree Foundation, London.
Beresford, P. and Croft, S. (1990b), 'A Sea Change', *Community Care*, 4 October, pp. 30-1.
Bryman, A. (1989), *Research Methods and Organization Studies*, Unwin Hyman, London.
Buist, M. (1988), 'Illuminative Evaluation', in Lishman, J. (ed.), *Evaluation. Research Highlights in Social Work 8*, 2nd edn, Jessica Kingsley Publishers, London, pp. 72-81.
Carrier, J. and Kendall, I. (1986), 'National Health Service Management and the 'Griffiths Report'', in Brenton, M. and Ungerson, C. (eds), *The Year Book of Social Policy in Britain 1985-86*, Routledge & Kegan Paul, London, pp. 195-218.
Clare, M. (1988), 'Supervision, role strain and social services departments', *British Journal of Social Work*, vol. 18, no. 5, pp. 489-507.
Croft, S. and Beresford, P. (1989), 'User involvement, citizenship and social

policy', *Critical Social Policy,* issue no. 26, pp. 5-18.
Denzin, N.K. (1970), *The Research Act in Sociology,* Aldine, Chicago.
Department of Health & Social Security (1975), *Better Services for the Mentally Ill,* Cmnd 6233, HMSO, London.
Department of Health & Social Security (1977), *Joint Care Planning: Health and Local Authorities,* HC(77)17, LAC(77)10, DHSS, London.
Department of Health & Social Security (Central Health Services Council) (1978), *Collaboration in Community Care,* HMSO, London.
Department of Health & Social Security (1983a), *Health Service Development: Care in the Community and Joint Finance,* HC(83)6, LAC(83)5, HMSO, London.
Department of Health & Social Security (1983b), *Report of the National Health Service Management Inquiry,* HMSO, London. (The first 'Griffiths Report'.)
Department of Health & Social Security (1987), *Promoting Better Health: The Government's Programme for Improving Primary Health Care,* (White Paper) Cm 249, HMSO, London.
Department of Health (1989a), *Working For Patients - The Health Service: Caring for the 1990s,* (White Paper) Cm 555, HMSO, London.
Department of Health (1989b), *Caring For People: Community Care in the Next Decade and Beyond,* (White Paper) Cm 849, HMSO, London.
Department of Health (1990), *The Care Programme Approach for People with Mental Illness Referred to Specialist Psychiatric Services,* HC(90)23, LASSL(90)11, DoH, London.
Department of Health (Social Services Inspectorate) (1991a), *Approved Social Workers: Developing a Service,* DoH, London.
Department of Health (1991b), *The Health of the Nation: A Consultative Document for Health in England,* HMSO, London.
Department of Health (Social Services Inspectorate)/Scottish Office (Social Work Services Group) (1991), *Care Management and Assessment: Summary of Practice Guidance; Practitioners' Guide;* and *Managers' Guide,* HMSO, London.
Evans, N., Kendall, I., Lovelock, R. and Powell, J. (1986), *Something To Look Forward To: An evaluation of a travelling day hospital for elderly mentally ill people,* SSRIU Report No. 15, Portsmouth Polytechnic, Portsmouth.
Fisher, M., Newton, C. and Sainsbury, E. (1984), *Mental Health Social Work Observed,* George Allen & Unwin, London.
Glennerster, H., Korman, N. and Marslen-Wilson, F. (1983), *Planning for Priority Groups,* Martin Robertson, Oxford.
Griffiths, Sir Roy (1988), *Community Care: Agenda For Action. A Report to the Secretary of State for Social Services,* HMSO, London. (The second 'Griffiths Report'.)
Guba, E.G. and Lincoln, Y.S. (1981), *Effective Evaluation: Improving the Usefulness of Evaluation Results Through Responsive and Naturalistic Approaches,* Jossey Bass, San Francisco.

Guba, E.G. and Lincoln, Y.S. (1989), *Fourth Generation Evaluation,* Sage, Newbury Park, California.

Hammersley, M. and Atkinson, P. (1983), *Ethnography: Principles in Practice,* Tavistock Publications, London.

Hampshire Social Services Department (1986), *Referral (Process) Survey - Draft Report,* (unpublished).

House of Commons Social Services Committee (1985), *Second Report: Community Care, With Special Reference to Adult Mentally Ill and Mentally Handicapped People,* HC 13-1, Session 1984-5, HMSO, London.

Hugman, R. (1991), 'Organization and professionalism: the social work agenda in the 1990s', *British Journal of Social Work,* vol. 21, no. 3, pp. 199-216.

Huxley, P. and Fitzpatrick, R. (1984), 'The probable extent of minor mental illness in the adult clients of social workers: a research note', *British Journal of Social Work,* vol. 14, no. 1, pp. 67-73.

Huxley, P., Korer, J.R. and Tolley, S. (1987), 'The psychiatric 'caseness' of clients referred to an urban social services department', *British Journal of Social Work,* vol. 17, no. 5, pp. 507-20.

Iles, P. and Auluck, R. (1990), 'Team building, inter-agency team development and social work practice', *British Journal of Social Work,* vol. 20, no. 2, pp. 151-64.

Isaac, B., Minty, E.B. and Morrison, R.M. (1986), 'Children in care - the association with mental disorder in the parents', *British Journal of Social Work,* vol. 16, no. 3, pp. 325-39.

Jones, K. (1988), *Experience in Mental Health: Community Care and Social Policy,* Sage, London.

Jones, L.R., Badger, L.W., Knopke, H.J. and Coggins, D.R. (1983), 'The emerging role of the primary care physician in the care of the chronically mentally ill', *Journal of Public Health Policy,* vol. 4, pp. 467-83.

King's Fund Institute (1987), *Promoting Innovation in Community Care,* Briefing Paper 3, King's Fund Institute, London.

Kingsley, S. and Towell, D. (1988), 'Planning for high-quality local services', in Lavender, A. and Holloway, F. (eds), *Community Care in Practice: Services for the Continuing Care Client,* John Wiley & Sons, Chichester, pp. 51-74.

Korman, N. and Glennerster, H. (1990), *Hospital Closure: A Political and Economic Study,* Open University Press, Milton Keynes.

Lavender, A. and Holloway, F. (eds) (1988), *Community Care in Practice: Services for the Continuing Care Client,* John Wiley & Sons, Chichester.

Marris, P. (1986), *Loss and Change,* 2nd edn, Routledge & Kegan Paul, London.

McKee, L. (1988), 'Conflicts and context in managing the closure of a large psychiatric hospital', *Bulletin of the Royal College of Psychiatrists,* vol. 12, no. 8, pp. 310-19.

McKeganey, N.P. and Bloor, M.J. (1981), 'On the retrieval of sociological

descriptions: respondent validation and the critical case of ethnomethodology, *International Journal of Sociology and Social Policy*, vol. 1, no. 3, pp. 58-69.
McKeganey, N. and Hunter, D. (1986), ''Only Connect': tightrope walking and joint working in the care of the elderly', *Policy and Politics*, vol. 14, no. 3, pp. 335-60.
Miles, A. (1987), *The Mentally Ill in Contemporary Society*, 2nd edn, Basil Blackwell, Oxford.
MIND (1983), *A Common Concern*, MIND Publications, London.
Ministry of Health (1962), *A Hospital Plan for England and Wales*, Cmnd 1604, HMSO, London.
Ministry of Health (1963), *Health and Welfare: The Development of Community Care*, Cmnd 1973, HMSO, London.
Mittler, P. (1987), 'Staff development: changing needs and service contexts in Britain', in Hogg, J. and Mittler, P.J. (eds), *Staff Training in Mental Handicap*, Croom Helm, Beckenham.
National Health Service Health Advisory Service/Department of Health Social Services Inspectorate (1989), *Report on Services for Mentally Ill People Provided by the Portsmouth and South-East Hampshire Health Authority and the Social Services Department of Hampshire County Council*, HAS/SSI(89)MI.485.
Øvretveit, J. (1986), *Organisation of Multidisciplinary Community Teams*, BIOSS, Brunel University, Uxbridge.
Øvretveit, J., Temple, H. and Coleman, R. (1988), *The Organisation and Management of Community Mental Health Teams*, Good Practices in Mental Health/Interdisciplinary Association of Mental Health Workers, London/Guildford.
Parlett, M. and Hamilton, D. (1972), *Evaluation as Illumination: A new approach to the study of innovatory programs*, Centre for Research in the Educational Sciences, University of Edinburgh, Occasional Paper No. 9, Edinburgh.
Parlett, M. and Hamilton, D. (1977), *Introduction to Illuminative Evaluation*, Pacific Soundings, Cardiff-by-the-Sea, California.
Parlett, M. and King, J.G. (1971), *Concentrated Study*, Research in Higher Education Monograph No. 14, Society for Research in Higher Education, London.
Patmore, C. and Weaver, T. (1989), 'Measures of Care', *Health Service Journal*, 16 March, pp. 330-1.
Patmore, C. and Weaver, T. (1991), *Community Mental Health Teams: Lessons for planners and managers*, Good Practices in Mental Health, London.
Phillips, D., Barritt, A., Booth, T., Jones, D., Lightup, R., Matthews, J., Melotte, C., Pritlove, J. and Simons, K. (1988), 'Classifying psychiatric crises: problems of reliability in post-coding open-ended questions', *Research, Policy and Planning*, vol. 6, no. 1, pp. 1-6.
Powell, J. (1991), *The Sevenoaks Club: A Joint Initiative in Day Care*, CEDR,

Department of Social Work Studies, University of Southampton, Southampton.
Powell, J. and Lovelock, R. (1987a), *Northern Road: A study of developing services for drug misusers*, SSRIU Report No. 16, Portsmouth Polytechnic, Portsmouth.
Powell, J. and Lovelock, R. (1987b), 'The role of consumers' views in the evaluation of services: a case study - the travelling day hospital', *Social Services Research*, vol. 16, no. 1, pp. 16-29.
Powell, J. and Lovelock, R. (1989a), *Cosham Mental Health Service Evaluation: Interim Report*, Department of Social Work Studies, University of Southampton, Southampton.
Powell, J. and Lovelock, R. (1989b), 'The development of community based adult mental health services - a research contribution', *Bulletin of the Royal College of Psychiatrists*, vol. 13, no. 12, pp. 662-6.
Powell, J. and Lovelock, R. (1991), *An Evaluation of a Developing Community Mental Health Service*, CEDR, Department of Social Work Studies, University of Southampton, Southampton.
Powell, J. and Lovelock, R. (1992), 'The development of community based adult mental health services - implications for professional practice', *Bulletin of the Royal College of Psychiatrists*, vol. 16, no. 2, pp. 73-5.
Ramon, S. (1985), *Psychiatry in Britain: Meaning and Policy*, Croom Helm, London.
Ramon, S. (1988), 'Community Care in Britain', in Lavender, A. and Holloway, F. (eds), *Community Care in Practice: Services for the Continuing Care Client*, John Wiley & Sons, Chichester, pp. 9-25.
Richman, A. and Barry, A. (1985), 'More and more is less and less: the myth of massive psychiatric need', *British Journal of Psychiatry*, vol. 146, pp. 164-8.
Ritchie, J., Morrissey, C. and Ward, K. (1988), *Keeping in Touch with the Talking: The community care needs of people with mental illness - a research study carried out on behalf of the Birmingham Community Care Special Action Project*, Social and Community Planning Research, London.
Sedgwick, P. (1982), *Psycho-Politics*, Pluto Press, London.
Smith, G. and Cantley, C., with Ritman, V. (1983), *Pluralistic Evaluation: A Study of Day Care for the Elderly Mentally Infirm (Summary Report)*, Department of Social Administration, University of Hull, Hull. (Note: A brief summary by the authors may be found in *Community Care*, 18 August 1983, pp. 20-21.)
Smith, G. and Cantley, C. (1985), *Assessing Health Care: A Study in Organisational Evaluation*, Open University Press, Milton Keynes.
Smith, G. and Cantley, C. (1988), 'Pluralistic Evaluation', in Lishman, J. (ed.), *Evaluation. Research Highlights in Social Work 8*, 2nd edn, London, Jessica Kingsley Publishers, pp. 118-136.
Soni, S.D., Steers, L., Warne, T. and Sang, W.H. (1989), 'Multidisciplinary teams and line management: practical problems and areas of conflict in

clinical psychiatry', *Bulletin of the Royal College of Psychiatrists*, vol. 13, no. 12, pp. 657-61.
Towell, D. (1985), 'Health and social services relationships in the reform of long term care. Giving impetus to local service development', *British Journal of Social Work*, vol. 15, no. 5, pp. 451-6
Wing, L. (1989), *Hospital Closure and the Resettlement of Residents: The Case of Darenth Park*, Gower, Aldershot.